Carole and FJ speak from their own personal story, compelling readers to walk with them through the unexpected storms brought on by invisible disabilities. Their story is both encouraging and heartbreaking. This couple's honest and vivid storytelling will challenge you to be more empathetic and compassionate toward friends and strangers.

—Dr. Nancy L. Potter
Ph.D.; CCC-SLP; professor and specialist in
neurologic disorders in the Washington State
University Elson S. Floyd College of Medicine and
fellow survivor of an invisible disability

Sunbreaks in Unending Storms is a book written from the heart and from the heart of experience. Join FJ and Carole on their compelling journey of ups and downs, battles and triumphs, tears and joy. Find hope, help, and healing through their experiences, wisdom, suggestions, and a faith in God that has withstood the test of time and the force of the gales of invisible disability.

—Francee Strain
Author, *No Ordinary Invitation;*
member of invisibly disabled community

FJ and Carole have welcomed us into their home and lives, as they honestly share the realities of life with chronic illness. Their story is real, their experiences as carer and patient need no embellishments. Chronic illness affects every area of their lives, yet their story is full of hope and practical tips to live the best life possible. This book is a must read for anyone living with chronic illness, caring for someone who does, or for concerned "observers" who know others in this situation.

—Sam Moss
Internationally known chronic illness advocate; creator and owner of the website and podcast *My Medical Musings*; writer for the website The Mighty; founder of the Facebook group Medical Musings with Friends

Sunbreaks
in Unending Storms

Understanding Invisible Disabilities,
How to Thrive There, and
How to Help

Carole Griffitts | FJ Griffitts

This publication is meant as a source of encouragement for the reader, but it is not meant as a substitute for professional counseling, nor does it constitute medical advice, diagnosis, or treatment recommendations. Always seek the advice of a trained counselor, physician, or other qualified provider with any questions you may have regarding a medical condition or treatment.

ISBN: 978-1-7369817-0-2 (ebook)
978-1-7369817-1-9 (paperback)
978-1-7369817-2-6 (hardback)

Dedication

We lovingly dedicate this book to our parents

Martin and Pauline Griffitts
and
Charles and Ruth Reader

who by their lives implanted in us
the eternal good news.

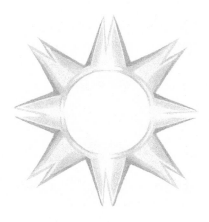

Contents

Acknowledgments   xiii
Foreword   xv
Explaining the Storms—An Introduction   xvii

Part 1
Sun and Storms—Our Story

1. Sunny Days in the Rose Garden:1966–1978   1
2. Cataclysmic Storms Oct. 1978–Sept. 1980   11
3. Tempests, Squalls, and Sunbreaks: 1980–1989   23
4. Drizzles, Whirlwinds, and Cloudbursts: 1990–Present   39
5. Damage Assessment—What Life Looks Like Now   55

Part 2
Navigating the Storms—Living This New Life

6. Weather Disturbances Everywhere—Other
   Families' Stories   73
7. Storm Consequences—Practical Responses   87
8. Turbulent Weather Impact—The Collision of
   Emotions   103
9. Stormy Transitions—Acceptance and New Purpose   119
10. On the Scene—Family   131
11. Responders—Medical Community   147
12. The Disaster Relief Team—Helpful People   161
13. Storm Observers—Friends and Onlookers   173
14. Why Storms Exist—Spiritual Questions   189
15. When Storms Get Personal—Spiritual Applications   203

Part 3
Responding to Storms—What You Can Do

16. Watching Others' Storms—How You Can Help   223
17. Navigating Your Stormyland—Tips for You   233
18. Living Stormy Lives—Summing Up the Storms   243

How to Know God—As Easy As A-B-C   251
Glossary of Medical Terms   255
Endnotes   263
Recommended Resources   269
About the Authors   271

"For I know the plans that I have for you,"
declares the Lord, "plans for welfare and
not for calamity to give you
a future and a hope."
Jeremiah 29:11

Blessed be the God and
Father of our Lord Jesus Christ,
the Father of mercies and God of all
comfort, who comforts us in all our
affliction so that we will be able to
comfort those who are in any affliction
with the comfort with which we
ourselves are comforted by God.
2 Corinthians 1:3–4

FJ's Tribute to Carole

There was a little Texas gal
Who came to California and found a special pal.
With lovely hair of gold and eyes of blue
My heart to her she drew.
Two hearts so in love
This kind is from God above.
Now as much of life has passed
Through storms of health that last and last
But God's comfort's here even in the stormy blasts.
But the time has come
My dear love, let us look at what God has done.
Two blessed joys, our sons
Their delightful wives into the family have come.
Seven precious grandbabies from heaven sent
We pray daily their hearts to God's will be bent.
At last my life's companion, eleven there are
To love, pray for, and adore
As forward, we tread the way to heaven's shore.

Thank You, Lord, for this wife I love
She has meant more to us
than family or friend can ever know
she has suffered more pain than her body did show.

Thank You, Abba,
the lovingest wife You gave
You sent from heaven to earth below

From me to you, Carole—
Your loving husband, FJ.

Carole's Tribute to FJ

Twelve short years.
Twelve years to walk side-by-side with you, FJ.
Twelve years to select activities using any criteria.
Twelve years to engage in energetic activities.
Twelve years for ordinary social interaction.
Twelve short years of normal family life.
And then the storms . . .

FJ, we had a great marriage for those first twelve years. Over forty years of storms have transformed it into an awesome union. Your love has been tried severely and found to be pure.

Our life has not turned out as we envisioned it. Too many years
of pushing my wheelchair when we should have been walking side-by-side,
of leaving me at home while you attended meetings, shopped, or went to our sons' functions alone,
of undertaking my responsibilities,
of doing so many "little" things for me,
of standing helplessly by while I endured unfixable pain.

Yet you stayed close to God, remained faithful, and retained your sense of humor. You supported and enabled me to keep on keeping on.

Our life has not always been pain, though. We have two exceptional sons and two awesome daughters-in-law. And now, seven incredible grandchildren. Wonderful extended families and warm friendships. Shared memories of beautiful vacations.

Thank you, FJ, for our life.
Thank You, God, for FJ.

Acknowledgments

We thank Wes and Bonnie, without whose encouragement this book may never have been finished.

We especially appreciate the effort Wes and Bonnie, Judy, Nancy, and Hank spent in reading the manuscript and offering suggestions.

Our special gratitude extends to Jayme and Richard, Jean and Andy, and Kathy for their willingness to be interviewed. We did not realize how intrusive the interviews would be. Thanks also to Tracee, her children, Eliza and Daniel, and her mom, Alma, for their input. Thank you all so much because your contributions added value to this work.

Audrey Griffitts, our granddaughter, provided the interior drawings. Thank you.

Jen Kline, of Line of Hope Creative, designed the perfect cover. Thanks, Jen, for your creativity. So many have offered positive comments on the cover.

Pam Lagomarsino, of Above the Pages, edited this book for us, but any errors remain our responsibility. Thank you, Pam, for your patience.

Jody Skinner, of Skinner Self-Publishing Services, formatted this edition. You took so much time to answer our numerous questions. You went above and beyond in editing. Thank you, Jody.

And our biggest thanks go to God, our Creator—the One who sustains us. Without Him, this book would not exist.

Foreword

The human experience is a frequent focus of commentary for fiction, poetry, and prose. That we all share experience but with endless variety of our own stories adds meaning for what it means to be human and drives us to learn from and about one another. Physicians are afforded a special privilege of viewing the human condition through the experience of our patients' humanity interacting with their daily, and often, long-term struggles in various states of health and disease. Working with people who struggle with nervous system disorders is an especially unique way of seeing the nature of an individual's personal narrative.

My experience with dystonia perhaps more than any other type of medical, neurological, or even movement disorder bears witness to what it means to be human and live daily with a condition that works against the ability to muster up movements of one's own free will. Involuntary twisting, turning, tremor, spasms, aches, and pains may all be part of the disorder of dystonia. The slow onset, protean patterns, and seemingly random triggers for worsening only add to the mystery people living with dystonia must learn to accept to some degree as a part of their new daily life. Even after a diagnosis of dystonia is made, this is often cold comfort to tell a friend or acquaintance the diagnosis—only to feel reassured by some clarity of diagnosis but have its name never before seen or heard by those who would seek to support.

It is with great enthusiasm that we now may approach these personal stories of those living with dystonia and other invisible disabilities. A brief glimpse into a short period of life recounting the initial symptoms, challenges with diagnosis, and breakthroughs and set backs of treatment shared with family, friends, and those who would be interested to learn more.

—Jason Aldred, MD FAAN
Neurologist; Selkirk Neurology, PLLC; Inland
Northwest Research, LLC; Clinical Assistant
Professor, University of Washington Department
of Neurology and Washington State University
School of Medicine

Explaining the Storms—An Introduction

Storm [stawrm]
"A disturbance of the normal condition of the atmosphere, manifesting itself by winds of unusual force or direction, often accompanied by rain, snow, hail, thunder, and lightning, or flying sand or dust."

—"Storm," dictionary.com

Kristy stood forlornly, staring out her living room window, not seeing the gorgeous view of sloping lawns leading to green hillsides beyond their apartment complex. She enjoyed a short respite from her pain and weakness that enabled her to stand for a few minutes, but she was so tired of being tired. She desperately wanted to take part in life and care for her family again.

Her multiple sclerosis seemed to be winning the war as she recalled ambulance rides to the hospital. However, Kristy remained unaware of how the campus community gossiped and said she was faking her illness. If she had known, she would have wondered, did those people think she wanted to be stuck in her house twenty-four hours a day? Did they believe she deliberately chose to ignore her children? Or that she would treat her student-husband that way? Couldn't they under-stand she didn't live this way by choice?

Welcome to the world of invisible disabilities. A disability is an impairment substantially limiting one or more major life activities. Invisible means unseen or indiscernible. This world of invisible disabilities has over twenty-three million American inhabitants.[1] If assembled in one location, this population would be equal to that of Florida in the United States. These people could define their lives as living amid ongoing storms with times of turbulence that come and come . . . and come, varying only in their intensity and timing. Kristy's story represents the heart-ache many people face daily. Although we only knew Kristy by reputation—and that long before Carole's storms began—we empathized with her situation, never realizing it would become our own.

Meteorological storms come in all shapes and sizes. Some are mild, bringing renewed life to the earth, while others bring cat-astrophic damage. Most fall somewhere between these extremes.

As with the weather, events can disturb our normal life con-ditions. Many of us will endure a disruption during our lifetime, ranging from mild and temporary to catastrophic and perma-nent. Unemployment and bankruptcy. Relationship problems and divorce. Grief and death. Chronic illness and debilitating physical difficulties. *Sunbreaks in Unending Storms* deals with this last type of event, likening it to storms in the lives of those with an invisible disability. Many principles presented here also carry over to other types of upheavals.

Unending storms occur in a place we call "Stormyland."

Welcome to Stormyland

Who is affected? Invisibly disabled people and those with chronic illnesses, a group we call *storm dwellers,* live in Stormyland. Their families and caregivers also dwell there. Stormyland affects another group of people we call *storm observers*—those who live outside these disturbances of physical challenges but see the turmoil. They visit, occasionally or often, to befriend and help those who live there. Wealth, level of education, and age—none matter. Residence can be in the United States or another country. In short, Stormyland can disturb anyone—rich and poor, educated and uneducated, old and young, and Americans and international residents.

What is Stormyland like? Stormyland differs for each person according to the specific disability. Unexpected thunderstorms, a forecast hurricane, or even a surprise flood-producing torrential rain can occur. Countless dreary times. Some rainbow days. Even a few sunny seasons. But always another storm to come.

When will it end? Most people's storms are transitory, although some last longer. But for the storm dweller, the prospect of inclement weather will never end. Chronic illness expert Marcus Brown shares a truth that also applies to unseen disabilities. "Chronic illness rarely responds to a direct intervention, and by definition, is elusive of cure."[2]

Where is it? Anywhere and everywhere.

Why does Stormyland happen? Sometimes, bad choices by an individual or someone else cause these storms. Other people were born that way. At times, microbes cause it. But in many cases, we never know why.

Storms can be unpleasant experiences—even disastrous—interrupting our plans. Yet, in the natural world, rains also serve beneficial purposes. They water the earth, producing crops, grass, flowers, and trees. Tempests often radiate a beauty of their own. Peace following the winds is pleasant, even if only by comparison.

We all realize that severe storms cause extensive damage and require years of recovery. So also, in a person's life, harm from repeated health-storms causes life-altering losses. These frequently recurring storms seem to last forever, and one wonders if life will ever be sunny again.

In this book about turbulent times, we strive to encourage, strengthen, and support storm dwellers by sharing our experiences and offering helpful suggestions. To storm observers, we provide information about dwellers' lives and ideas and tips on how to help them. Underlined terms found throughout the book appear in the glossary where additional details can be found.

Introduction to Invisible Disabilities

Defining disabilities can be daunting. The <u>Americans with Disabilities Act of 1990</u> (ADA) states, "An individual with a disability is defined as a person who has a physical or mental impairment that substantially limits one or more major life activities, a person who has a history or record of such an impairment, or a person who is perceived by others as having such an impairment." To qualify for Social Security benefits—most people's definition of *being disabled*—a person must be unable "to engage in any substantial gainful activity."[3]

Others define disability more loosely. "A person is considered to have a disability if he or she has difficulty performing certain functions (seeing, hearing, talking, walking, climbing stairs and lifting and carrying), or has difficulty performing <u>activities of daily living</u> [ADL], or has difficulty with certain social roles (doing school work for children, working at a job and around the house for adults). A person who is unable to perform one or more activities, or who uses an assistive device to get around, or who needs assistance from another person to perform basic activities is considered to have a severe disability."[4]

However, not all disabilities are disabling. "Many living with these challenges are still fully active in their work, families, sports, or hobbies. Some with disabilities can work full or part-time but struggle to get through their day, with little or no energy for other things. Others are unable to maintain gainful or substantial employment due to their disability, have trouble with daily living activities, and/or need assistance with their care."[5]

Now add an unseen element to disabilities, and you have *invisible* disabilities. Sherri Connell, a co-founder of the Invisible Disabilities Association, is an expert in the field because of her experiences. Her insights help people understand the concept: "The term invisible disability refers to a person's symptoms such as extreme fatigue, dizziness, pain, weakness, cognitive impairments, etc., that are sometimes or always debilitating. These symptoms can occur due to chronic illness, chronic pain, injury, birth disorders, etc. and aren't always obvious to the onlooker."[6]

An invisible disability is not a mental illness, psychiatric condition, or imagined. Nor is it hypochondria or laziness. It is real. Just because doctors can't find a cause or others can't perceive it doesn't mean there is no problem. (Please realize that while an unseen disability may not be caused by mental or psychiatric issues, a mental illness or psychiatric disorder qualifies as an invisible disability.)

In this book, we limit ourselves to dealing with unseen chronic conditions severe enough to affect a person's participation in normal life activities.

Invisible Disabilities Lifestyle

Take a virtual tour of Stormyland. Come along and consider your reactions to the following questions.

- How would you cope with all-consuming, incapacitating physical struggles that you know, short of a miracle, will never end during your lifetime?

- Could you live with a future of unpredictable, progressively worsening symptoms?
- How could you continue visiting doctors who couldn't diagnose these problems?
- What would your feelings be when you could no longer do life's ordinary activities?
- How would you raise your children if you couldn't do what parents are supposed to do?
- Would you still enjoy your grandchildren if you couldn't share in their activities?
- Could you maintain your relationship with a loving God who would allow you to go on hurting?

Now you have briefly lived in a virtual Stormyland. What do you think of it? Unfortunately, these circumstances—and many others—occur all too frequently for those undergoing lifelong storms.

The following tempestuous scenes exist for many storm dwellers. Can you empathize with them? Can you help?

Situation #1: You can do your job adequately, but accomplishing every task is beyond your ability. Because you appear normal, your coworkers look askance at you. Can you survive emotionally?

Situation #2: You tell a good friend you are too fatigued to attend that two-hour conference with her, and she answers, "Well, I'm tired, too, but I'm going anyway." You know ignoring your fatigue will cause pain for several days or even weeks, but she doesn't understand. Will you lose her friendship?

Situation #3: You love God deeply, yet you continue to suffer from a debilitating chronic disease. How do you feel when you hear stories of other people being healed, and friends tell you to just have faith?

Situation #4: Your spouse, who assists in your activities of daily living, needs serious surgery. Now, what do you do?

Situation #5: You live in pain most days, so how would you respond when an extended family member denies your distressing reality?

Situation #6: You live in severe pain every day, but no relief exists. How do you face it?

Everyone has a deep, heartfelt desire to be understood, but people with hidden limitations often encounter misunderstanding, unbelief, and rejection. Thus, we offer you—the observers—information about living in Stormyland and tips and suggestions for helping and supporting your friends. For you dwellers, we want to aid your journey by offering insights for coping and enduring. We invite all of you into our lives and those of other families to witness examples of living in this turbulent world.

The Invisible Disability Difference

What is so different about living with invisible disabilities? Times of suffering come to all as they experience four common types of adversity.

The largest group includes temporary misfortunes expected to end. Flu. Heart surgery. A lost job. These difficulties—some minor, some severe—will eventually resolve. Invisible disabilities will not.

Sudden-onset events resulting in permanent loss constitute a second form of adversity. Death of a loved one. An accident which causes quadriplegia. These difficult conditions share with invisible disabilities the "forever" component; however, these permanent losses neither improve nor worsen while invisibly disabled individuals often face capricious and degenerative changes.

Persons experiencing a terminal illness make up the third kind. Coping with those circumstances involves a special skill set not needed in the other types.

A fourth category of adversity exists: it has no definitive beginning and no ending and is often unpredictable and progressive.

Invisible disabilities fall into the fourth group. Living with those difficulties differs significantly from the other three because of their nature. Consequently, coping and acceptance require alternative approaches. Information in many books written and sermons preached about suffering is incomplete or doesn't apply. These authors and preachers often present insights that fall short of the reality of life with endless, imperceptible impairments.

Although all four groups experience many of the same emotional difficulties, spiritual questions, and relationship issues, individuals with unseen limitations encounter additional problems. They associate with people who don't realize, or may even disbelieve, their problems are real, which brings added distress and complications. Furthermore, these people spend years seeking a diagnosis and treatment, often encountering doctors who won't accept the reality of their symptoms. They cry out for people to understand why they live such limited lives.

By the close of this book, you will better understand what living with invisible disabilities is like, how it differs from other situations, and how you can lighten someone's load. If you live in storms, we trust you will find hope to persevere and new tools to accomplish that.

Stormyland Residence

Each year, viewers see news clips of massive tornado damage. During a 2017 broadcast, one man reported a tornado had just begun to lift his mobile home when a tree fell on the trailer, keeping it from being pulled up into the storm. Even when an imminent warning sounds, insufficient time may exist for people to escape. We wish warnings could be given days before a tornado strikes. We want to see signs around the impact area, saying, "Danger! Keep out! Tornado at work!"

Some health problems are so destructive doctors might label them stealth-tornado-storms. Health issues that pull strength from randomly affected individuals can be as terrifying as colossal storms. We share with you Carole's story of life in an unending health-tornado and how it has affected our family.

Health-tornadoes are sneaky, their arrival time hard to pin-point. Carole's tornado came subtly, beginning with a seemingly insignificant physical occurrence in 1978. Only days later, a cataclysmic storm hit. What did Carole think after her first—and worst—injury: severe back-muscle damage? Would she recover? What was her future? How did her family feel and react? What about her friends? FJ imagines these injuries as caused by a Silent Stalker, a caricature of evil. He visualizes this unseen personage as it stalks, pursues, and attacks many unsuspecting people today.

In 1984, at age thirty-seven—six years after her initial injury—Carole finally received her first answer: a lifelong condition, possibly worsening. The rest of her life? That equaled forever! Only thirty-seven, married, with boys ages thirteen and sixteen, this appeared a daunting prospect. What would we do? What should we think? How could we face such a life sentence? And we had no idea it would get worse nor that more diagnoses were yet to come. Our story illustrates the realities of life in Stormyland.

Spiritual Perseverance

We want dwellers and their families to know God does care and provide. We have learned that even though turbulent times may last a lifetime, peace, comfort, and solace can be found in God's promises.

God is the firm foundation of our lives. Without Him, we don't believe we would have survived this life—at least not successfully. We want to share the comfort God has supplied for weathering our storms. At times, our coping skills weren't equal to the awfulness we faced, but Almighty God always provided the strength and encouragement we needed to persevere.

People undergoing troubles crave understanding from someone who will comfort them during these stressful, stormy trials. Few people are willing to come alongside; they want to care but rarely have enough time or compassionate patience to show it. Caring people need empathy and tenacity to dig into the depth of pain individuals with permanent, yet imperceptible, difficulties face twenty-four hours a day, seven days a week, three hundred sixty-five days a year. Yet, our God of compassion fully knows our spiritual, mental, and physical struggles and provides for our needs.

Peace is a coveted commodity sought by people throughout the ages. This quote from Henry Drummond speaks of rest, but to us, it conveys peace during times of turmoil.

> Two painters were asked to paint a picture illustrating his own idea of rest. The first chose for his scene a quiet, lonely lake nestled among mountains far away. The second, using swift, broad strokes on his canvas, painted a thundering waterfall. Beneath the falls grew a fragile birch tree, bending over the foam. On its branches, nearly wet with the spray from the falls, sat a robin on its nest.[7]

Jesus, in John 14:27, tells us, "Peace I leave with you; My peace I give to you." As this robin found rest in a noisy, wet environment, so we too can find peace in God during blustery weather.

The darkness of Carole's storms can't hide the light Jesus shines in our life. Friends' concern and love from family reflect that light. It shines in the quality of her medical care. It shows in the way He lifts our spirits. Jesus' light shines as He becomes her safe haven of retreat when things are too awful to bear. Even as far back as 1987, Carole's words spoken to Ione Baptist Church reveal her desire to trust Jesus. "He [Jesus] means to me, first, that I willingly give an 'okay' to whatever He allows to happen in my life, even if it is (and continues to be) painful. That was a hard lesson for me to learn because I don't want to hurt. I want to be strong again." So, do we believe God to be trustworthy or not? We answer with a resounding "yes!" We agree with Paul, who said in 2 Corinthians 4:16 (MSG), "So we're not giving up. How could we! Even though on the outside it often looks like things are falling apart, on the inside, where God is making new life, not a day goes by without his unfolding grace."

Sneak Peek at Sunbreaks in Unending Storms

- Part One relates the forty-year journey of one person, invisibly disabled, living in never-ending, cascading storms. Carole and her family exemplify how unusual symptoms can be and how difficult life can become with progressive, unpredictable difficulties. We seek to bring understanding to people who have a family member, friend, or acquaintance who suffers from invisible disabilities.
- Part Two uses our experience and that of three other families to show how people can prevail even during storms. We examine four areas of struggles storm dwellers face: practical, emotional, relational, and spiritual. Also, we want storm observers to realize the complications and extra burdens that people with unnoticeable impairments and their families face. We include tips and practical ideas for dwellers and observers.
- Part Three summarizes *Sunbreaks in Unending Storms*. A chapter for compassionate observers recaps suggestions and ideas to help dwellers. The chapter for dwellers draws together hints and helps to aid in the journey through Stormyland. The conclusion sums up Stormyland.

After reading about our experiences, you may find them to

be weird and implausible. Others' stories may seem strange and improbable. Please suspend your judgment and believe their veracity. We need your acceptance.

Still, sometimes dwellers can be their own worst critics. In the early years, Carole experienced some days when she felt good, with only mild pain or weakness. At those times, she assumed the weird bouts of pain and weakness must be her fault. Was she lazy or making it up? She didn't truly think so. Nevertheless, when another challenging event occurred, she knew with certainty she bore no blame. We hadn't known about <u>neurological</u> issues nor the difficulties of diagnosing them. If Carole had known anyone who experienced similar problems, she might have supposed the person to be lazy, a little crazy, or a hypochondriac. Carole realized that at times she had accused herself of all these things.

We tell of our odyssey of increasing, ever-changing disabilities: how we've succeeded, how we've failed. We incorporate lessons we've learned and questions we had—both answered and unanswered. We include practical issues we dealt with and how others helped—or how we wish they'd helped. And we explore the spiritual ramifications of healing not received.

You probably already realize we are not trained medical professionals. FJ is retired; Carole is disabled. We are parents and grandparents. We have friends. We love experiencing nature. But none of these gives us the training to give you medical advice. What we do is share experiences of those living with invisible disabilities. If you need help, please get advice from a trained professional.

Come along as we share our story of weathering forty years of living with Carole's brain disorders. Before cataclysmic storms hit, we lived a typical life: marrying and starting a family, pursuing a career, enjoying recreational activities, and carrying out everyday tasks. "Sunny Days in the Rose Garden" gives you a glimpse into the normalcy of our family's early years.

Part 1:

Sun and Storms—Our Story

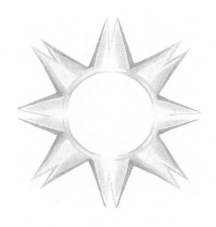

Chapter 1

Sunny Days in the Rose Garden:
1966–1978

The basics of growing roses:
ensure plenty of sunlight; avoid very exposed, windy sites;
use the right amount of watering.

—"The Basics of Growing Roses,"
David Austin Roses

*As Gomer Pyle used to say, "Surprise! Surprise! Surprise!"
Exactly right, FJ thought. He saw Carole walking across the lawn
in front of the campus dorm, hurrying to the office to sign out for
her date with an Air Force man she would soon meet—him! He
saw that beautiful young college student and considered her the
most alluring woman the good Lord ever made. She had shoulder-length hair like silky golden sunlight. What an intriguing
vision, he concluded. A prayer flitted through his mind: "Lord, I
think marrying her would be absolutely wonderful. Could this possibly
be the woman of my dreams? Is this love at first sight?"*

FJ Reminisces

Meeting and Dating

My Air Force roommate and his fiancée arranged the first date for Carole and me in September 1965. We double-dated, enjoying a movie. That intriguing evening began a lifelong journey, sharing hopes and dreams of our deepest, most precious longings. She became the person of my most intense interest.

More evenings and times together formed a bond of love that grew into a relationship of permanent commitment. After just two months of getting to know each other, we quickly became inseparable. Soon, I asked Carole to marry me; this lovely and very intelligent woman, sporting a giant smile, honored me with a resounding yes.

We talked of varying subjects like family, faith, and our future as husband and wife during these times. My world became incomplete when she was on campus for class and I was on duty with the Air Force. Our commitment's strength was soon tested as the Air Force sent me on a temporary duty assignment five thousand miles away. For six months, we flooded the mail with love letters. I looked forward to those perfume-scented letters from Carole because they reminded me even more of her. Our time apart seemed to last forever, but finally the months of separation ended. After I returned to the good old USA, we agreed on a wedding date of July 16, 1966. We planned for my father, the Reverend James M. Griffitts Sr., to preside over our ceremony. Remembering those days of our delightful romance produces a desire for an ability to relive that part of life.

Getting Married

Oh! Happy days were here at last as our day to marry drew near! The Air Force had approved my leave time. I began the four-hundred-mile drive from Mather Air Force Base, near Sacramento,

California, to Carole's home in Carson, California, where the ceremony would occur.

I speculated the miles seemed to have had road lengthener applied in massive quantity, many times over, for they passed so slowly. Why did the hands on my watch never appear to move? What did that blinking red light on that black and white vehicle in my rearview mirror mean? I thought I remembered hearing such a thing indicated a person should pull to the roadside and see if that driver needed assistance. So, I did, but the man said, "You were really hauling the mail back there." In nice, formal handwriting, he offered me an invitation to appear in court or pay a donation to California.

For the rest of the trip, the road appeared even longer, with the miles passing still slower. When I got to Carson, I discovered this country boy wasn't a proficient city navigator. I called Carole from somewhere around a waterfront to get clearer directions to her house. Finally, I arrived at her home, and we were at long last united again.

July 16, our long-awaited wedding day, arrived—the beginning of our life together. We received many presents, but the best gift has been what we vowed before God: "For better or for worse." To put this another way, "No matter what may come, I promise before the Lord my God to stay with you. I will be a spiritual support as well as a material provider to the best of my ability. I will do this till death separates us." We didn't know how severely these vows would be tested in the coming years.

Commitment and faithfulness are lifelong endeavors that result in a satisfied state of mind. Honoring marriage vows and remaining loyal is more important for a peace-filled soul than houses or bank accounts. We did not realize how some marriage values, deeply embedded in our spirits, were to influence the direction of our life. As years passed, applying the priorities of God first, family second, and church third grew ever more important. Marriage is more than just a man and woman lovingly devoted to living life as husband and wife; it should be, ought to be, can be a couple united in God's purpose.

Carole's parents and mine faithfully taught us Scripture as they raised us in homes where they modeled the Christian faith. Psalm 127:1 speaks to establishing family life: "Unless the LORD builds the house, they labor in vain who build it." Looking back, we can see how we applied this verse to our marriage and raising our sons.

Raising Sons

At the end of my Air Force enlistment in 1968, our rose garden expanded when Tom joined our family. What a sunny day! This healthy baby boy favored us by sleeping the whole night through at six weeks. This rose garden enlarged again in 1971 while I was in college when Bill brought even more sunshine into our lives. And he surprised us by sleeping through the night at three weeks! Tom and Bill have bestowed countless blessings on us through the years.

Bill and Tom both displayed outstanding intellectual ability from the earliest age. Tom was a good-natured, happy child. Focusing on completing whatever task he began has been one of his most salient traits. Bill was a bubbly, joyful child with a dash of reckless daring. As a bee flits from flower to flower, Bill quickly went from one activity to another. They each exhibited a surprising sense of humor even as young children. Tom's expressed itself in a droll manner, while Bill's conveyed wit and whimsy.

Seminary—graduate school for ministers—followed college. During those seminary days, Tom's humor evidenced itself one Sunday when I preached in a small church nearby. After services, a couple invited our family to their home for lunch. As our hosts and Carole and I sat around the dining table talking,

4

we repeatedly heard a screen door slam. The husband recognized the commotion's cause as a person and said, "Stop that!" The noisemaker, four-year-old Tom, replied, "It's not me. There's a herd of woodpeckers out here."

Bill displayed his daredevil spirit when, at four years of age, he thought it would be fun to ride his tricycle down a steep hill. Of course, there are no brakes on a kid's trike, and that ride resulted in a crash, permanently cracking a front tooth.

Tom loved to build. He constructed towns, bridges, and other creations with his Tinkertoys, Lincoln Logs, and Bridge and Girder set. Outside, he used Tonka toys (metal construction vehicles, such as dump trucks and graders) to work in the dirt.

Although Bill, too, liked to build, he preferred learning how things worked by taking them apart. He also loved Tonka toys, especially crashing his dump truck by letting it freewheel down rough hills.

Being read to during his early years, then later reading for himself, was one of Tom's favorite activities. He had all his books memorized, so woe to us if we skipped a page; he insisted we read it. Wiggly Bill never favored reading, although he would listen to short books. Their favorite books also evidenced personality differences: Tom preferred *Green Eggs and Ham*; Bill favored *Where the Wild Things Are*.

Each son's strengths played an important part through the years as they made many adjustments to Carole's disabilities, but that is a story for the future.

Living Life

After seminary, I began my career as a pastor. A family of four seemed a good fit for the calling I knew came from God: pastoring small rural churches. Such work offered meager monetary provision, so more children would have been a financial burden. We welcomed family life even on a limited income. Great good can result from having few possessions: family members can focus more on personal relationships, resulting in closer bonds.

Evenings were always a fun family time, playing games, reading, or watching television. Devotions consisted of reading from a children's Bible, singing a song, and saying prayers. We were poor but a happy family who partnered together in life. Training Tom and Bill for age-appropriate tasks and teaching them to take responsibility for themselves played an important part in our parenting. Working with the boys provided fun times and offered teaching opportunities. When bedtime approached, we all sat on the floor, putting away Lincoln Logs, blocks, LEGO bricks, toy cars, and plastic airplanes—and whatever other toys they'd played with. As Tom and Bill matured, they became more self-reliant because they'd learned personal responsibility.

I remember many varied household tasks Carole and I shared. It seemed we both changed a million diapers. And in those days of non-disposable diapers, you rinsed them, flushed away the contents, and put the cloths in a diaper pail until a washer load accumulated. We spent most Saturdays working as a couple, washing our car and pickup and doing other household chores. Two working as one accomplished work easier and faster. Time passed quickly as we enjoyed the camaraderie of being together.

What a good and wise choice I made to fall in love with Carole because she proved to be a natural, helpful editor of my required college writing. Since my high school graduating class had only thirteen students, my education lacked preparation for college. No matter that she graduated high school in a class of six hundred students, she would still have been a genius in scholastic matters. I wrote well, and she edited well, and in January 1973, I received a bachelor of arts degree.

In 1978, just two years before I was to graduate from seminary, my beloved wife began experiencing physical pain and weakness. This woman had been so strong that, together, we could move a couch with a heavy hide-a-bed. Now, she entered a storm of unending pain and increasing weakness. The rose garden was no longer so free of thorns. Although we were never blessed financially, we had enjoyed and been thankful for good health, two wonderful sons, and the blessing of knowing God as Savior for eternity.

Carole Remembers

FJ successfully captured the fun-loving spirit of our early years that we call sunny days in our rose garden. As FJ asserted, we used to wistfully say, "We may not have much money," but then happily add, "At least we have our health." Little did we know we would only have twelve short years to say that! For less than one-quarter of our marriage, we would live a traditional lifestyle. However, we turn that around and say, "At least we had that long!"

Remembering the Early Years
We lived like any other young couple with small children, experiencing sunshine and showers. Roses grew wonderfully, and the occasional thorns were just part of living. We spent a typical life working, shopping, attending church, spending time with extended family, and savoring life. We played with, disciplined, taught, and treasured our sons during those early years.

Our family loved our frequent visits to grandparents and siblings. Tom and Bill enjoyed visiting with their cousins, exploring the houses and yards, and inventing games. Both sets of grandparents and several uncles and an aunt lived close enough for weekend visits. Tom and Bill appreciated seeing their grandparents, and even their great-grandparents and great-aunts and great-uncles.

From the time our sons were old enough to take part, our family enjoyed outdoor activities. FJ and I came by our love of

7

nature effortlessly since he grew up in the Redwoods of Northern California and my family frequently camped. We all walked in our neighborhoods and along nature trails while the boys were still young. Camping came later because we didn't own a tent until they were older. Once we acquired one, we camped frequently. We loved observing and experiencing nature's beauty.

It was just an ordinary day when Tom, Bill, and I hurried from the mall back to our car. Bill was four, but he, being tired, did not want to rush. So I picked him up, put him on my hip, and rushed out with Tom to our car. This standout memory stays with me because only three years later, lifting even ten pounds proved to be beyond my ability! I miss those sunny rose garden days.

During these years, our family faithfully attended Sunday School, worship services, and other church activities. As a teen, FJ had experienced God's call to be a pastor; his circuitous route just took sixteen years of adventure to get there. First, FJ joined the Air Force a few months after high school. Two years into his enlistment, we met and married and began our family. FJ strongly desired to further his education, and he sensed a pull to be a military chaplain. After finishing his Air Force commitment, he attended college and completed his four-year degree in three. Then came seminary to begin the three-year master of divinity degree, which took seven. FJ and I both worked, sometimes full-time, sometimes part-time, to support our family.

We detoured along the way, taking breaks from school to work. We lived in four different states in those seven years. FJ and I moved ourselves each time, sometimes with help from family. With each move, we expectantly looked forward to a better future. But then we always returned to school.

Recalling My Health
Throughout these sunny years in our rose garden, my health seemed as normal as anyone else's. Even though I experienced

8

several unusual and isolated neurological issues, no one thought anything could be seriously wrong. I considered them to be "strange" things many people undergo. Neither the doctors nor FJ and I supposed these episodes to be worrisome or harbingers of serious things to come.

While living in Santa Rosa, California, in 1977, I experienced multiple episodes, even more odd. A <u>neurologist</u> wanted to do a neurological workup, but I let others guilt me out of it. They blamed me for what was happening and said I shouldn't waste the doctor's time. They caused me to believe I was imagining problems. What might my later life have looked like if I had followed through with the neurological testing?

We excitedly returned to seminary for the third time, knowing FJ would finally finish his degree. He began his pastoral ministry in a rural town in Washington State in 1980—two years after the storms started. We would have done well to consider James 4:13–15 when planning. "Now listen, you who say, 'Today or tomorrow we will go to this or that city, spend a year there, carry on business and make money.' Why, you do not even know what will happen tomorrow. What is your life? . . . Instead, you ought to say, 'If it is the Lord's will, we will live and do this or that.'" Even though we weren't pursuing education to make money, we proved the truth people do not know what the future holds. Planning is good, but flexibility is crucial when surprises arise.

We had not realized that September 1978 was the last time our family would live a normal life; storms of pain and weakness that had unleashed their ferocity would continue for years as disturbances of varying degrees of intensity. Although these tempests of disabilities affected only me, those same weather disturbances impacted all four of us. The foundations of a happy, stable, fun-loving family, which we had laid in our sunny rose garden, prepared us well for the future.

Chapter 2

Cataclysmic Storms
Oct. 1978–Sept. 1980

Pecos Bill, that fabled cowboy of unique roping ability, had been granted miraculous power over nature. Yep! He roped and subdued a cantankerous weather phenomenon known as a tornado. These twisters are unpredictable—no knowing when or where they will strike nor what mischief they will bring on structures or people. Suddenly taking a wild dip down out of the sky wreaking catastrophic havoc in previously peaceful lives, tornadoes live up to their alarming reputation. Who can envision the destructive impact of such a storm?

—FJ Griffitts

Lunch break at last! In a place with incomparable natural beauty! Golden sunshine. A radiant blue sky. White puffy clouds slowly floating along. Gentle ocean breezes. A delightful day. Two secretaries strolled through the seminary campus courtyard to the stone bench sheltered beneath an olive tree. There they enjoyed lunch along with friendly conversation.

Carole, the blue-eyed blonde with shoulder-length hair, wore a blue peasant-style blouse. Suddenly, she felt stinging on her bare right shoulder. Startled, she exclaimed, "Ouch! That stings!" Were they sitting underneath a beehive in the tree? They could see nothing. Repeatedly surprised, she continued exclaiming, "Ouch!" More stings. "Oh well. Just one of those things. No big deal," she thought.

The whispers of discomfort she experienced that day would shortly turn into a whirlwind of pain that would shatter her life of normalcy. Pain and physical disability would buffet her. Ah! Where was a medical Pecos Bill, one with the power to subdue the oncoming pain, turn it back, and eliminate its source? Gentle winds preceding a tornado can be withstood, but what about the turbulent winds that follow?

Little did FJ and Carole realize this idyllic day with the odd, slight pains signaled the approach of a raging storm that would soon be unleashed in their lives. Even less did they realize these bouts of pain, weakness, and exhaustion would come and go for the rest of her life.

Carole's Recollections

The first storm struck with little warning; a few wisps of mist were our only hint that forever-changes loomed ahead. The first few clouds went unrecognized as harbingers of disaster. For days following that lunch, stings reoccurred all over the right side of my back. We could find no discernible cause, no means of prevention, and no way to predict them. Blessedly, each stinging pain lasted but a moment.

Unusual, darkening clouds gathered, but still, we didn't recognize the cataclysmic storm coming. Only a few days later, a Thursday, that whole side of my back hurt badly. Friday, it was worse but still bearable. That weekend, even with the pain, FJ and I continued with our plans to attend a church conference for Sunday School teachers at a retreat center. Sitting unsupported at the campfire became difficult and painful but still doable.

On Monday, lightning flashed, thunder boomed, winds howled, and clouds of catastrophe burst. Nonetheless, we remained unaware of coming severe consequences. After working for a few hours, hurt became pain, so I visited the doctor who came to the seminary twice a week. She prescribed over-the-counter pain medication and sent me back to work. By my next visit a few days later, my pain had become unbearable and work intolerable. She prescribed alternating between the maximum dosages of <u>acetaminophen</u> and aspirin every three hours. She sent me home for complete bed rest. Her diagnosis? I had torn every back muscle on my right side, from under my shoulder blade to my waist and from my spine to my side. The doctor had no idea what caused this very strange injury.

This first storm had broken in all its fury, permanently altering our family's life.

The Stormy First Year Begins

FJ had just returned to Golden Gate Baptist Theological Seminary in Mill Valley, California, to finish his master of divinity. I worked full-time at the seminary's library in the technical services department. My job involved various repetitive movements, required lifting heavy card catalog drawers, and necessitated frequent bending. Our older son, Tom, was ten, and our younger son, Bill, seven. We lived with my parents twenty miles away while we waited for a campus apartment to become available. Since we planned to move shortly, we enrolled our boys in a Mill Valley school. Each morning, we all headed to the campus where FJ studied, I worked, and Tom and Bill attended school. Until the clouds burst.

Soon after the deluge hit, an apartment became available. FJ and the boys moved our household goods, a few at a time, while I stayed at my parents' home on bed rest. Each morning, they took whatever fit into our station wagon along with them to

Mill Valley. Severe pain prevented me from even holding a knife to make our sons' sandwiches. When I could sit long enough to tolerate riding to Mill Valley, I joined them for the trip, resting in our apartment during the day. I could do absolutely nothing to help unpack boxes or arrange furniture. I had to lie there helplessly and watch as others did my work. This was the first such happening but, sadly, not the last.

Extreme pain filled that first three weeks; it even hurt to take a deep breath. I spent that time lying on my back—except for necessary car rides, getting up to eat, and seeing my doctor weekly for evaluation. After three weeks, she saw a slight improvement. Several months later, I could sit up long enough that she cleared me to work one hour a day. As I strengthened, I gradually lengthened that time, but months passed before I could work full-time.

Three months after injuring myself, under my doctor's supervision, I began exercising at an infinitesimally slow pace. Moving carefully, I would lower myself to the floor and lay down. First came a successful completion of one pelvic tilt! Next, by tucking my feet under our old-timey radio cabinet and gently pulling up my upper body, I completed my first partial sit-up! My workouts began with one repetition a day of each exercise, duplicating this for three days. When that was easy, repetitions increased to two. I followed that pattern, persevered, and nine months later was doing twenty repetitions.

Gradual increases and careful movements defined my physical life after that cataclysmic storm.

Life Changes the First Year
That incredibly tough year, all four of our lives changed. FJ had to do duty as a student, part-time wage earner, and househusband. For months, household chores fell to him and the boys. As my condition improved, I slowly began to help. After a month, I set

the table for meals—four knives on one trip to the table, forks and spoons after that, plates next, and glasses last. My ability to do housework gradually improved, but it still seemed as if I could do virtually nothing. Tom and Bill attended school, but they also had extra household chores. Emotional pain resulted from being unable to take care of the boys and the house as I had previously. Working as much as possible and resting my back most of the remaining time filled my days. Healing occurred but at an agonizingly slow rate.

"If you feel bad, just keep on working. If something needs doing, just keep on keeping on and get it done!" We often heard those or similar words that first year. However, we quickly discovered the fallacy of that sentiment. Some injuries require rest to heal. Others recur if you continue the causative activity. We realized you sometimes can't just push yourself. Working when your muscles have reached their limit causes increased pain and injury, requiring longer healing time.

Rain diminished; winds calmed down; the storm assaulting my body finally ceased. By the end of twelve months, I had regained ninety-five percent of my function. Even though my doctor still didn't understand why the injury had occurred, we believed this had been a one-time storm. We assumed that when my back healed, pain and hard times would be just a bad memory. That belief sustained us, helping us survive the first stormy year.

And Then . . .

By October 1979, I could work full-time again. And then, once more, another raging storm hit. Same work activities. Same injury. Same doctor. Same healing approach. But, a different outcome.

There was to be no full recovery this time. However, recognizing the need for medical intervention and rest more quickly reduced the severity of that second onslaught. We used the same medications and rest. We attempted the same exercise regimen.

15

Yet, we only saw partial healing. The same exercises proved too difficult for my strength. Rest helped little. The cause still stymied doctors. Yet again, our family experienced a substantial impact.

I saw a physical therapist that spring who taught me to pay attention to my activity and notice when the pain recurred. By using that approach, we finally identified work tasks as the culprit. The repetitive arm movement put more pressure on my back than it would tolerate, and it reacted in severe muscle spasms. Doctors still couldn't understand why my body wouldn't bear the stress so many others at that job had easily withstood. Several years passed before we thought we had the answer.

Throughout those two years, dealing with my out-of-control situation of spasms, pain, weakness, fatigability, and imperceptibly slow improvement discouraged us. Yet, because we believed it to be a one-time (two-time?) occurrence, we experienced little anger, despair, or fear. Because we expected to see an end to storms, we didn't have spiritual questions that arise when one suffers from an unending condition God chooses not to heal. However, significant emotional and practical issues resulted from my injuries. I don't know what FJ or the boys remember, but I imagine they often dealt with a short-tempered, whiny mom. Frustrations ensued from being unable to do tasks I considered my responsibility. Pain and weakness made it difficult to be kind and attentive, let alone cheerful. But we survived intact as a family, and we expected good times to return.

My work had taught me time-management lessons that proved invaluable in years to come. Working in library technical services was all about prioritizing. There were always jobs to do. Some work demanded immediate attention, while other projects could be ignored for a time, and many jobs fell in between. Sometimes we had to ignore tasks that clamored for our attention while working on those without a deadline. Otherwise, we would never have found time to work on less important tasks. To accomplish this, we needed the opportunity and ability to break large projects into small parts.

During this time, I learned to prioritize personal work and segment larger projects. My job had also trained me to overlook activities that could wait or, worse, that I could no longer do. I learned the necessity of prioritizing all those jobs just begging for my attention. I mastered the skill of putting aside pressing tasks to work on less urgent jobs. I learned to cut a big project into small parts and work on it over several days or weeks, realizing I'd eventually finish. Using my downtime in my recliner to plan and organize prepared me to work when uptime came.

Still to Come

FJ would graduate in June, and we assumed he would be a church pastor soon after that. We also presumed our storms would cease because the job-related strain on my back muscles would stop, and life would return to normal. Even after this second round of disabilities, we still believed it to be a temporary, albeit long-lasting, situation. In September 1980, FJ received a call to be the pastor at Ione Baptist Church in northeast Washington.

God-inspired coincidences happened. That month, FJ and I received a card from a friend with Jeremiah 29:11 written on it. When we studied our Sunday School lesson for that week, we discovered the same verse there. Then we read a daily Bible reading based on Jeremiah 29:11. We reasoned, "Lord, You must be trying to tell us something. Does this mean our storms are over?"

"'For I know the plans I have for you,' declares the LORD, 'plans to prosper you and not to harm you, plans to give you hope and a future'" (NIV) became my life verse as I realized unpleasant times didn't cause lasting harm, and I could have hope. However, at the time, we interpreted Jeremiah 29:11 to mean the storms were over. Little did we know over thirty years of suffering would pass before we understood the real answer.

FJ's Memories

Years of Carole's unrelenting pain seemed like a science fiction story, starring Carole and an invisible malicious alien being who indiscriminately caused <u>lancinating</u> pain in unsuspecting people. The following is a narrative of Carole's life as I remember it.

This being we call the Silent Stalker noiselessly pursued the woman who had no knowledge of the unending storms he would unleash in her body in the years ahead. No visible visage could be observed as he lurked near this wife and mother of two young boys, but now she suffered painful, cutting, stabbing effects from his power to bring bedeviling debilitation. This stranger was without any form, yet Carole became unpleasantly aware of his presence. Just thirty-one, she had been—and always would be—an ambitious, intellectually gifted woman. She had enjoyed a good life with normal physical ability since her recovery from polio at two years old. This Silent Stalker intruded into her physical well-being, altering who she was and was to become. A sometimes frightening life was about to begin for Carole—an unending storm of unpredictable physical hurt.

This scene became our reality; it was the most alarming portrayal of harm entering a life that one might imagine. Her sudden onset of pain from an inexplicable cause was daunting. As any person suffering would, she hoped for relief, yet extreme discomfort disturbingly continued. Even in the awfulness, sometimes when Carole suffered intense pain, I saw and felt a divine nearness as her countenance appeared to glow. Likely, this glow was due to blood pressure or medication, but God's presence was and is her real comfort. Still, seeing her in such intense pain, I grieved for her in my inmost self.

Before the Storms
Who was this mother and wife? What had she done to deserve

this onslaught of weakness and physical torment? If she had known the intense pain to come, what would she have done? She was happily married to a ministerial seminary student. She worked in the campus library, where her wonderful aptitude for technical tasks well suited the work. Our sons were just seven and ten.

The year was 1978, and the seminary was located on Strawberry Point near Mill Valley, California, just five miles north of the Golden Gate Bridge. A variety of bushes, trees, and lawns were visible from the library. When Carole looked out her office window, she viewed the campus grounds and housing situated on rolling hills. Below the campus grounds lay an inlet from San Francisco Bay; waters rippled by ocean breezes glistened in the sunlight. I can't remember seeing a place any lovelier than Golden Gate Seminary.

Life had been pleasant for Carole and me and our sons, Tom and Bill. We walked both on campus roads and along the roadway by the bay inlet. We dreamed about our future as we walked, imagining where we would live after graduation. One day on our stroll, I envisioned living in the mountains where there were lakes and trees. Never did either of us imagine an adversary was waiting silently to stalk Carole. We were happy with a simple life filled with purpose and good health while we focused on life's horizon in joyous anticipation of the future. Instead, a storm of pain and loss of physical strength lurked just ahead.

In October, Carole experienced cataclysmic back-muscle pain akin to a burning fire of torment. The extreme severity of the first onset of Carole's unending storm of physical disability lasted three months, followed by nine months of slow recovery. Nevertheless, the unseen Silent Stalker remained a lurking, shadowy, unidentified thing for many years.

Our New Tempestuous Life

This time demanded adjustments as the boys and I took up household tasks Carole ordinarily accomplished. I don't remember them complaining. They weren't prone to grumbling but rather were willing to do necessary work. One of the most helpful steps during this difficult time was to do whatever our strength enabled us to do, practicing the old proverb to keep going and putting one foot in front of the other.

For several weeks, Carole was completely helpless to do needed household tasks; it took most of the year for her to resume her normal activities. Tom and Bill helped me by setting the dining table, washing dishes, and taking out the trash. They were gofers, getting their bedridden mom a glass of water, fetching a book to read, or changing the television channel. As for me, I studied, worked part-time, cooked, laundered clothes, and supervised the boys. We must have been good parents to be blessed with two awesomely helpful sons.

During these tough times, reading the Bible or remembering a Scripture verse created a wellspring of strength, hope, and endurance. We kept in mind what a pastor friend once said: "We ought to pray without ceasing and not cease without praying." We came through this terribly hard season, spiritually and physically helped by God and His people.

Carole has always enjoyed worshiping in private and with others at church. We attended services in Santa Rosa, forty-five miles north of Golden Gate. We traveled through beautiful green hills along Highway 101, seeing farms and small towns along the way. Just off the freeway, we spotted cattle grazing contentedly in lush, green pastures. We observed many stands of eucalyptus trees scattered over the countryside. Altogether, a refreshing journey each week.

Before the disabling storms, Tom, Bill, Carole, and I savored our family time on the hour's ride to church each Sunday. We played games, caught up on weekly happenings, and enjoyed the changing scenery of the seasons. At church, Tom and Bill each attended their Sunday School class. Carole and I went to our Bible classes: Carole to teach third-graders and me to lead senior adults. We joined up again for the worship service. After church, we traveled another fifteen miles to visit my grandmother for the afternoon.

These good times ended with the onset of the calamitous storms, which meant Carole could no longer endure the car trip. Tom, Bill, and I continued attending church by ourselves for the next three months. After that, Carole could again accompany us by reclining her car seat to ease pressure on her muscles. She used that time to do isometric leg exercises, seeking to regain strength.

Storm Breaks, Rainbows, and More Storms

Storms have interludes of calm even if these breaks include more pain than vibrant health. The pause when ongoing hurt ceases and pain relents is so greatly welcome. After a short or long siege of incessant pain, these breaks reminded us of the advertisement asking, "How do you spell relief?" Carole answered, "I HAVE NO PAIN." Between the first onset of the baffling medical mystery and the second episode, a blessed period of calm existed, lasting over the summer. Carole had regained most of her strength.

Loving these sunbreaks and rainbow days during the summer of 1979, we journeyed to Yosemite National Park in the Sierra Nevada Mountains to explore the trails, waterfalls, lakes, and trees. Towering mountains rose 7,000 to 13,200 feet. The streams, pools, lakes, and hiking trails made a fascinating adventure into nature's wonders. Tom, Bill, Carole, and I enjoyed hiking and tent camping. Tom and Bill climbed large rocks and a tree here and there. The boys and I floated on the Yosemite River's refreshing icy-cold water on a hot summer day. The four of us hiked to see backcountry beauty as Carole could still walk long distances

21

unaided. Of course, the activity kept our appetites alive and well for Carole's cooking skills to quell. Even though Carole still felt pain at times and hadn't regained her full strength, she reveled in the outdoor living. These times of family fun and enjoying each other have been a most fulfilling gift of life.

The severe back-muscle pain recurred in October 1979, and life for us never returned to a normal family situation. A cure has yet to be found to destroy the insidious invader. Carole, the boys, and I longed for a medical cure to restore her to an active, healthy life. My wife was and is excessively curious about nearly everything on the planet. So during the coming years, she began searching for an answer to this problem that continued to baffle the medical community, and her, and our family for nearly four decades.

The adversary had taken her strength and ability to fulfill the tasks of wife and mother she had enjoyed doing since our marriage and our sons' births. For so long, she physically couldn't be out of bed except for extremely short times. If only we could have known a Medicine Woman (you remember that television series?) would come along, we would have cried out, "Where the heck is that Medicine Woman?" Just a jest, but amidst physical hurt, mustering a smile or laugh at the silly has been a balm of encouragement.

During the early years of her physical distress, we—the boys, I, and our Carole—thought she would eventually recover her health. No way did our minds ever consider this would become a permanent part of life. We lived with expectant hope for the healing we knew would release Carole from her physical throes of pain.

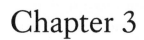

Chapter 3

Tempests, Squalls, and Sunbreaks: 1980–1989

"The typical example [of a sunbreak] is of sunlight shining through a hole in cloud cover. Artists such as cartoonists and filmmakers often use sunbreak to show protection or relief being brought upon an area of land by a receding storm."
—"Sunbreak"; Wikipedia

In 1984, the doctor delivered his life-staggering diagnosis: "You have post-polio syndrome." Carole responded, "How long will it last?" He answered, "The rest of your life, barring a miracle. Of course, if a miracle happens, don't turn it down." That summer, while vacationing at FJ's parents' home in California, Carole walked down the long driveway to sit under a tree by the brook as she sought solitude, contemplating her "forever" prognosis. "It will be for the rest of your life" echoed in her thoughts. Would it truly never end? She believed she could not face a lifetime of limitations. She cried.

FJ Journals

That insidious Silent Stalker had briefly been held in check from causing Carole further physical pain storms. This respite brought freedom from her grinding back pain. During this reprieve, her leg, arm, and hand strength neither decreased nor increased. Nevertheless, ongoing residual effects caused by her previous episodes remained. Despite the physical damage she had suffered, this was a time of relief when she didn't cry out from stinging, stabbing, cutting pain. Carole enjoyed a welcome interlude of freedom from further debilitation. Later, her health would continue to spiral downward.

In times without storms, she joined in family activities. During these occasional <u>remissions</u>, she could still cook wonderfully. When sunbreaks and rainbow days occurred, we walked the short distance to our city park, where we sat on a swing and watched the Pend Oreille River flow past as we pleasantly chatted about life. Short mountain drives just minutes from home were times of delight as we looked down on the river meandering through the verdant valley.

Life at Ione
Carole could again drive our car for long distances. In September 1980, she drove our AMC Matador station wagon while I drove our old Chevy pickup and trailer one thousand miles on our move from Mill Valley, California, to the small town of Ione, Washington.

This lovely valley in Washington's northeast corner is nestled among evergreen-forested mountains. Our biggest surprise occurred that fall when the tamaracks—coniferous trees we assumed to be evergreens—burst forth in flaming yellow colors. For fourteen years, we reveled in God's creation of this exquisitely beautiful corner of the Northwest. It never ceased to fill us with wonder. What a wonderful treat in life—except for times of unending rain or winters so long they never seemed to end long enough for summer to happen.

Amazingly, during the first winters, Carole joined our sons and me in enjoying cross-country skiing. Just a twenty-minute drive brought us to groomed ski trails to engage in this exhilarating activity. At twenty-five degrees, skis slid easily over the crusted snow, and we savored beautiful scenes of a deep blue sky above a forest of trees tufted with pristine white snow. The woods glistened with the beauty of winter. Ice crystals drifted downward, gleaming like floating diamonds in the sunlight.

In Ione, our family enjoyed pleasant years as our sons grew from boyhood to young adulthood. When we arrived, Tom was in junior high and Bill in elementary school. Carole coached our sons in their studies, providing encouragement and guidance. Both were gifted students, soon proving their academic ability. Their intellectual capacity still impresses me. Eventually, they left us with an empty nest. Tom earned a master's degree while serving in the military. Bill is a Certified Public Accountant. I'm thankful and proud of these wonderful sons God blessed us with.

A standout day for my family and me happened in 1984 when I was commissioned as a First Lieutenant (Chaplain) in the US Army Reserve. I had the privilege of serving God in the Reserves for the next sixteen years. Each time we moved, a nearby unit needed a chaplain.

Sunbreaks and Rainbow Days
Yearly vacations were times of travel, seeing nature's beautiful places. Recalling camping in state and national parks evokes nostalgic memories of joys our family shared. One of my favorite recollections was of our earlier camping trip in Yosemite National Park when Carole could still hike unaided and fix our meals.

Our Yellowstone National Park trip remains an outstanding

memory. We delighted in hiking the aesthetically pleasant forest and volcanic area trails. We oohed and aahed and wowed at scenes so unusually spectacular that we could find no intelligible words worthy of them in our vocabulary. Nature's abundant remarkable phenomena lured us into investigating and enjoying the fascinating sites. Mammoth Hot Springs was shaped as though landscaped with flat spaces, resembling steps carved in a rock cliff. Mineral colors drew us to gaze with wonder into numerous pools of water to see multicolored rocks beneath. Carole, in her wheelchair, the boys, and I viewed sights of geysers, hot springs, and bubbling mud pots. Scenic Blacktail Pond was encircled with a profusion of goldenrod flowers. In 1984, Morning Glory Pool's color was a mixture of deep sky blue and aqua teal. At that time, a boardwalk wide enough for a wheelchair encompassed this amazing treat of nature's alluring beauty.

People in wheelchairs can tour many of Yellowstone's natural wonders. We had rented a chair for this trip; shortly thereafter, we bought one. Our teenage sons pushed their mother in her wheelchair so she could see more scenic park attractions. We made some unlikely places accessible by one of us holding each side of her wheelchair and one pushing from behind. Using this method, we explored many fascinating attractions. We saw the great falls of the Yellowstone River. What a magnificent sight! Down a trail from Old Faithful Geyser, we saw rainbows transform Riverside Geyser into a uniquely beautiful scene, one among many.

A Short Respite
The old saying, "It never rains, but it pours," seemed to fit Carole's unwelcome medical adventures during these years. Unpredictable storms emanating from unknown causes produced unpleasant effects. Physical attacks continued, incrementally battering the health yet remaining to Carole.

We were cozy and comfortable in the house the church

provided to its pastor and family. Compared to our small seminary apartment, this eight-hundred-square-foot parsonage felt quite roomy. In this house, the Silent Stalker again pursued Carole as she periodically suffered more unidentified <u>neuromuscular</u> symptoms. Sometimes, I'd come home from pastoral duties, and she would be in a deep sleep, appearing unconscious. Carole calls these episodes "spells," which she explains later in this chapter. Other times, her sleep resulted from medication. The first medicine I recall was Amitriptyline, which caused her to sleep so much I thought she might be dying. She experienced varying amounts of pain mixed with weakness. For me, this onslaught of episodes was an emotional roller coaster. I began to think of her as being on a slow downward spiral, health-wise.

Tom and Bill may have unconsciously blocked out their awareness of the partial loss of their mother. They lost having her at their school sports activities. They lost her presence to enjoy hiking together as a family. They lost the clean house, pleasant meals, and delicious baking she had previously accomplished for them.

Help from Others

Again, our sons and I had more household duties to do, just as we had in seminary. During these years, church women came to help us. Twice, they came to spring-clean the house thoroughly and competently: Judy, another Judy, Helen, Deanna, Ann, and Lois. They were so good I thought perhaps they were angels in disguise. Lois lived a block away and often stopped in to see if Carole had any immediate need. Cathy lived behind the parsonage and often helped with cleaning and being a friend who cared enough to be there as company for Carole.

Some women cooked for us, especially at Thanksgiving. They baked desserts throughout the year. In Carole's worst year, Cathy even addressed Christmas card envelopes when Carole couldn't even sit up or hold a pen long enough to write the information.

Cathy, Ruth, and others helped Carole use her library skills to catalog the church's library.

More Losses

As the years passed, we both engaged in a battle of fearful apprehension as various ill effects would return. It was a vicious cycle: she would stabilize, then worsen again. But never would she improve. I thought the process seemed similar to an unstable chemical reaction. When her condition worsened, it would leave us with a sense of foreboding expectancy, contemplating what might come next. Where is the source? What can we do? Is this a harbinger signaling her death?

What a drastic difference in her life compared to when we first moved to Ione. Another remission was over. No longer was our family taking bike rides or going cross-country skiing. The Silent Stalker had begun again to torment the young woman. Pain came to different body parts, bringing intense weakness where there once was vigorous strength. No longer were her legs, arms, and back strong enough for heavy housework, such as vacuuming, sweeping, or dusting. She could no longer cook as much or as often.

This eventually led to a great promotion for me as I again became responsible for food preparation. Have you ever noticed Beetle Bailey often appeared by a large mountain of potatoes he had been tasked to peel? I could now peel potatoes as proficiently as Beetle Bailey because I had practiced sufficiently to become a veteran peeler—a reward for participating and not just merely observing. I also became an accomplished preparer of bacon and eggs. Hamburgers and more hamburgers, and maybe a gourmet Oscar Mayer hot dog created variety in my tasty menu. Boxed meals containing necessary ingredients also contributed to our menu.

What have I learned? Husbands, be warned: kitchen competence can cause your clothes to shrink. Why? Because if you create desserts, it's the cook's duty to taste them to be sure the delightful sweets are truly delightful. Oh, for the return of a twenty-nine-inch waist!

Carole Chronicles

Our New Life

In 1980, we assumed my pain and spasms would resolve in time, since I no longer worked. I'd be back to normal, able to be a wife, mother, and homemaker. Sadly, weeks turned into months and months into years. Our storms lessened from cataclysmic to frequent tempests and squalls, interspersed with days when winds died down, the rain stopped falling, and the sun shone. During these times, we lived the cliché "live, laugh, and love."

Even though I did everything right—rest, attempted exercise, and careful activity—no significant improvement occurred. Exercising to regain strength failed. Doctors did not understand why spasms would resolve but spontaneously recur. Since we presumed some action I performed caused these spasms, we spent years observing my actions, desperate to ascertain why. We expected discovering the action would enable us to modify movements and eliminate pain.

Meanwhile, the family adapted to reality: Mom couldn't do what other moms could. She still accomplished many light tasks as long as she exercised care in choosing what she did; even then, she often needed help.

I made up the term *tweener* to describe these years: neither fully disabled nor fully functional. For example, when I baked cookies for school lunches, I often needed help stirring the stiff cookie dough. Countless times, I'd start a job expecting it to be within my capabilities then discover I couldn't finish it.

There is a "darned if you do, darned if you don't" syndrome for people with invisible disabilities. If I husbanded my strength and rested properly, I looked as healthy as anyone else. When I didn't rest, I looked weak. I had to decide whether to take care of myself, which resulted in some people's disbelief, or to push myself beyond endurance so they could see something was wrong. Taking care of myself and feeling better seemed a healthier way to live, no matter what others thought!

On the Physical Side

At age thirty-seven, in 1984, I finally received a diagnosis: post-polio syndrome (PPS). This condition would never go away and would probably worsen. This "life sentence" equaled "forever!" In my thirties, married with two teenage boys—that was a daunting prospect. What do we do or think? How do we face a life sentence like this? And we had no idea life would get worse.

One conscious decision I made concerned my response to pain and weakness. These conditions predispose one to crankiness, whining, and complaining—unpleasant behavior for onlookers to endure. Although the problems were beyond my control, my reaction was not. Emotional outbursts only added to the unhappiness FJ and the boys already endured. It also affected any friends who visited. So, I strove for happiness despite my challenges. FJ and the boys will judge how successfully that strategy worked, but I tried hard not to allow my pain, fatigue, and frustration to boil over. The hardest struggle occurred at home: it was so tempting just to let my distresses erupt.

Weakness, fatigability, pain. The primary symptoms of PPS include weakness, fatigability, and muscle pain, all stemming from changes in polio-affected muscles. Swallowing and breathing issues also surfaced a few years later. I had contracted a light case of polio at age two and had seemed to recover completely. Through the years, though, I had noticed strange weaknesses that friends didn't have. Now those slightly weakened muscles deteriorated further. However, my symptoms never quite fit PPS.

It would be years more before we knew why. Years more before we discovered the reason for oddities like a twisted hand, making writing difficult yet allowing me to crochet.

One day, it came time to walk the quarter-mile to the post office and pick up our mail. And then—"Not again!" I wailed. I had sensed I was stronger, so the walking should have been fine; after all, I did it frequently. However, I tired too quickly, losing strength, and had to stop and rest. But I had plans! I couldn't afford the downtime!

Another day, I noticed our carpet needed vacuuming. Since I was feeling okay, I cleaned one small room. Since that went well, I vacuumed the living room. Then I thought, "Uh-oh. That was too much! I should have stopped with one room." By then, I was not only tired, but I also hurt! "It will take a week or more to heal this spasm." When compensating for weak arms while vacuuming, the large back muscles spasmed. Who would have suspected? Well, I should have. I didn't understand why, but I knew the process.

Fatigability is a symptom of neurological diseases where muscles weaken after even minor exertion and need time to resume their previous function. It remains my biggest problem. Fatigability is more than just tiring as the resulting weakened muscles cause muscle injuries.

Weakness, pain, and fatigability interact. Weakness produces painful spasms that can become injuries, which trigger more pain. Fatigability can hurt and often causes weakness. Pain can generate weakness, which begets fatigability.

Even more weakness. Although our family had enjoyed walks since the boys were children, we began serious hiking when they were teens. We enjoyed hikes of three to five miles. In 1980, we had climbed the two-and-a-half-mile Mount Lassen trail; it had an elevation rise of two thousand feet. Coming down taxed my strength to its utmost and only the thought of EMTs taking me

31

down the steep path kept me from quitting. My ability to walk leveled out for a few years, so we enjoyed moderate hikes. In the mid-1980s, again at Lassen, I did my last long hike of four miles; our sons had to support me on each side, half-carrying me, for the last half mile. After that, my ability to hike or walk decreased every year, from two miles to one to one-half to one-quarter, despite repeatedly trying.

Our camping adventures began with tents and sleeping bags, which we transported in our station wagon, along with the boys' bicycles on top. When I could no longer endure sleeping on an air mattress, we bought a camper. We added a lounge chair for relaxing outside. The wheelchair, which we began using in 1984 for "walking" long distances, became a fixture. I could do fewer and fewer camp tasks.

Grocery shopping meant spending all day in Spokane, two hours away. At home, I helped FJ bring groceries in and put them away. As time passed, I had to let FJ bring them all in but still had the strength to put them away. Fast-forward a few years more, and I would need to rest upon arriving home before helping.

In our early Ione years, I still walked through stores. A few years later, walking any distance became impractical. However, using a wheelchair didn't stop me from shopping. In grocery stores, FJ pushed a cart with one hand while pulling my wheelchair with the other. FJ experienced profound satisfaction with the debut of riding carts, exclaiming, "Hallelujah!" That spelled relief for FJ.

When I could no longer walk into a store, shop, and walk out again, we applied for a disabled parking permit. That experience brought mixed emotions: happy because it made our life easier; sad since it represented increased disability.

The time frame for the following snapshots was 1989, my weakest period. Frequently, when church time came, I thought I'd go that day, although I knew I could only stay for half the service

32

before severe weakness set in. Good thing we lived next door so I could walk home without bothering anyone. Another day as I designed a plastic canvas box for my friend, I became exhausted, and I had only been up thirty minutes. Now what? Other times when my downtime was finished, I was exhausted and couldn't get up and move around. What should I do? Still another time, the kitchen needed cleaning. That was my job; however, I was so tired, and I hadn't even done anything. Now, FJ and the boys would have to do everything—again. Why was this happening? Even doctors didn't understand. Why, God?

And then this time of severe weakness inexplicably ended, for which we praised God.

"Spells." "Where am I? What time is it? Where are my feet? Do I have my socks on? Ouch, my legs hurt. Oh, I must have had another 'spell.' This one was a doozy!" Such continue to be my thoughts when waking from a "spell."

A unique condition, which I (along with my doctors) call "spells," has plagued my life since FJ's seminary days. Every few years, the manifestations seemed to mutate, but the basic structure remained the same. All doctors believed they occurred, but none could diagnose them. As "spells" completely disable me, they have proved the toughest part of my life to cope with. FJ found them disconcerting as I appeared unconscious to him, and he wondered if I was dying. After so many occurrences, he knew that wasn't true, but my unnatural appearance still disturbed him.

My "spells" are episodes of paresis (partial paralysis). The severity of each episode determined how dysfunctional my limbs became. They followed a predictable half-hour-to-two-hour cycle. I often appeared asleep. They caused mild to severe leg pain and sometimes arm and head pain. After they ended, my muscles returned to their previous condition.

Thunderstorms and "spells" share a common theme. Certain conditions must exist for either to happen, and each can strike without warning, but specific occurrences of both are unpredictable. Circumstances develop that mean thunderstorms are probable; situations arise that make a "spell" likely. The only trigger I found was fatigue; it seemed to predispose me to a "spell" but not necessarily cause one. They recurred several times a week. They continue to this day.[8]

Daily Life

My days alternated between rest and activity. Uptime meant varying activities using different muscles, so some rested while others worked. Downtime meant resting on a daybed, not lying in bed nor sleeping. This relieved the pressure from my muscles—legs, arms, and trunk. Recuperating in the living area enabled me to remain part of the family and enjoy visitors. I read, watched TV, or interacted with family and friends. My talented husband designed and built the daybed.

I loved reading while reclining, but holding a book fatigued my arms. I developed a system for resting my arms while still reading. It used a lightweight board and two rectangular foam pillows. Rubber bands around the board held my book open while it rested on the bottom pillow and leaned against the top one, enabling me to turn pages easily. However, if the book were large or heavy, the rubber bands couldn't hold it. Through the years, I've made and decorated several sets of pillows and boards; they're inexpensive and easy to replace.

A typical day for me in the early years involved reclining for about an hour to relax the spasms, restore my strength, and return some endurance. Uptime meant three to four hours in mild-to-moderate forms of activity before losing strength and needing to recline again. By 1989, I averaged being down one hour and up one-half hour. As some strength returned, the time frame stabilized at one hour down and two hours up.

I loved an author's ideas about keeping track of the "what

and when" of symptoms. I decided to chart these daily. It only required a few minutes each day. These records, tailored to my needs, enabled me to dazzle doctors. They appreciated the details as it helped them make decisions.

Adapting and compensating became our family's way of life so I could carry out essential tasks and fun activities. I retained enough strength to perform activities of daily living (ADL), only occasionally requiring FJ's help. Frequently, FJ had to go to functions by himself. When we shopped, he had a choice: go in by himself or push my wheelchair. Vacations were modified to allow me to take part. FJ and our sons were willing and able to do this for me.

Problems abounded as we sought to adjust; mistakes happened. Overestimating my strength and underestimating the task remained my biggest challenge. FJ was much better than I at estimating my strength. He found it frustrating and discouraging to live with a beloved wife he couldn't help to feel better. It required patience and wisdom for him to parent, pastor, and oversee household tasks.

Spiritual Considerations

By 1987, it was painfully obvious that not only would my problems never end but they would also continue to slowly and progressively worsen. Spiritual questions abounded, some we still have no answers for. Meditating on special verses provided emotional relief. During the worst times, Psalm 69:30 brought comfort: "I will sing to the LORD as long as I live; I will sing praise to my God while I have my being." I could praise God no matter how weak I was. Psalm 104:33, which says, "I will praise the name of God with song and magnify Him with thanksgiving," reminded me my "being" would continue in heaven where I will praise Him forever.

Memorizing hymns also helped me cope, as did listening to

35

music. I sang songs while lying there inactive. "Holy, Holy, Holy" was one of my favorites to sing. Considering the endless skies of "Montana Sky" liberated my spirit to soar.

Extraordinary encounters. Two remarkable happenings occurred during these years. Today, they still epitomize my feelings about God and my suffering. His significance so transcends earthly experiences that anything He allows, for whatever reason, pales compared to who He is.

The first experience occurred while walking in Ione's city park. Upset concerning my prognosis, I talked to God about it. An imaginary scene ensued, involving a choice for me. If God healed me, but it wasn't His first choice for my life, would I accept it? Or would I accept the prognosis and trust God that His reason was good? It seemed as if God said He would heal me if I chose, but in doing so, I'd forgo His best plan for me. Let me be clear: I don't believe God causes evil, but I do believe He uses what we see as bad for good purposes. We just can't always see the good.

The second occurred at our church's Bible study on John's gospel taught by a visiting preacher. My fatigue and weakness were at their worst, so I attended in my wheelchair. Since the meeting was on the second floor, FJ had to carry the chair up a steep, narrow flight of stairs while I struggled up.

When Mary Magdalene encountered Jesus in the Garden of Gethsemane after the resurrection, she initially thought He was the gardener. However, she instantly recognized Jesus the moment He spoke her name. When the teacher reached the point of saying Jesus called Mary's name, my mind heard Jesus lovingly whisper, "Carole." Everything around me disappeared. My only awareness was of Jesus' presence. Neither the wheelchair nor my weakness nor my life's challenges mattered compared to Jesus knowing me. His love overwhelmed me as He spoke my name. All the storms no longer seemed important compared with who God is.

So, does my suffering make sense? No. Is it okay with me because of who God is? Yes. I know God is still good even if He never heals me. Isaiah 55:8–9 speaks of God's thoughts and ways being totally different than ours. Psalm 135:5–7 adds that God controls the storms.

Halcyon Days

Life wasn't all hard times. Our family enjoyed fun along the way, both in everyday living and on rainbow days.

A favorite time for our family was the Christmas season. We loved planning gift-giving, shopping for or making gifts, and wrapping them—and keeping secrets sometimes taxed our ingenuity. Christmas music played. In fact, FJ enjoyed Christmas music any time of the year. I began collecting manger scenes; to me, they expressed the essence of Christmas. Since I love light, combining manger scenes with candles was especially meaningful. I could glance up from reading and see the light of Christmas. The season has always meant so much to us because of Jesus' birth.

Living in northeast Washington afforded innumerable opportunities for seeing gorgeous scenery, hiking, cross-country skiing, fishing, and hunting. Days abounded with sunbreaks and rainbows, especially for FJ, Tom, and Bill.

Vacations involved travel and camping since our families lived in Northern California. Sometimes, we journeyed down the Oregon and California coasts, then back up through Central Oregon. Other times, we meandered our way down and back, traversing much of California and the Northwest. We camped in national parks, state parks, and national forest campgrounds. On day trips, we toured monuments and historical places with our families. When we toured the Oregon Caves, I was still walking, so I joined the guys. However, when we reached a flight of stairs, I balked. No way. Since our guide said they would come back down, I sat on the bottom step and waited, much to our guide's chagrin.

When we vacationed in Yellowstone and Glacier, we used a wheelchair for energy conservation, allowing me to see more sights. When we hiked, the guys pushed me as far as the chair would go. Leaving it by the trailside, I walked until my strength faded. I often wondered what other hikers thought about seeing an empty wheelchair in the wilderness. We explored British Columbia on our vacations. One time, sixteen-year-old Bill propelled himself in my chair around the camp loop, doing wheelies along the way. What looks he received! The wheelchair certainly added spice to our trips.

And Then . . .

We rode the good, the bad, and the ugly roller coaster of unpredictable pain, weakness, and fatigue during these years. Sustained, severe pain was rare, unlike the catastrophic injuries of 1978–79. This chapter of our life ended with Bill's graduation, leaving us with an empty nest. For the next fifteen years, days of drizzle and frequent wind and rain periods filled my life. And then, new, disturbing changes occurred as we experienced cloudbursts and whirlwinds and fewer clear days.

Chapter 4

Drizzles, Whirlwinds, and Cloudbursts: 1990–Present

"Drizzle consists of very small raindrops, larger than cloud droplets, but smaller than normal raindrops. It usually occurs when updrafts in clouds are not quite strong enough to produce rain."

—"What is Drizzle?"
weatherquestions.com

Diamond Lake nestles high in the Oregon Cascades mountain range. Campers relish its peace and beauty. In 1990, FJ and Carole relaxed in their campsite's privacy, loving the antics of nearby chipmunks. "Hey Carole, is your sweet tooth sending you a message that now would be a good time for an ice cream sandwich?" FJ grinned. "You bet," she laughed. Hopping on their bicycles, they traversed a steep uphill section of the bike trail and reached the store. Later, they cycled two miles along the level sun-dappled pathway leading to shady Noisy Creek, where they watched lazily flowing water.

Fast-forward a couple of years. They were delighted to find the same campsite available. However, this time, when getting ice cream, she had to push her bike up the trail's hilly part to the camp store. They still loved the ride to Noisy Creek.

Fast-forward again. Now, Carole couldn't bike to get ice cream.

Neither could she cycle the whole distance to Noisy Creek. FJ pushed her in the wheelchair to enjoy both these activities. It remained a soothing, relaxing place to camp.

Fast-forward to 1995. They now lived on the outskirts of Canyonville, Oregon. One joy they shared was short bike rides around the area. As Carole was too weak to pedal far, they added a small electric motor to her bicycle, allowing them opportunities for family fun.

These snapshots of FJ and Carole's life demonstrate the slowly progressive loss of strength Carole sustained during these years. Sometimes, the weakness arrived as a tempest; sometimes, as a squall portending bigger trouble. Occasionally, sunbreaks appeared, bringing respites of relief.

1990–2004

Sunbreaks and Rainbow Days

Carole: Despite dreary days of drizzles, gray days when fog rolled in, and still-too-frequent stormy times, sunbreaks and rainbow days occasionally materialized. Happy days we spent with our sons as they attended college. Intriguing days we met and became acquainted with our daughters-in-law-to-be. Sunny days when grandchildren entered our family. Even though my condition impacted all these relationships, each connection brought enjoyable interludes, reminding us of patches of blue sky amid dark clouds. Being with family enhanced these days.

We enjoyed family get-togethers at Thanksgiving and Christmas, sometimes at our house, sometimes at Tom's or Bill's. Memorial Day, the Fourth of July, and Labor Day saw our family barbecuing in our spacious yard. Graduations, baptisms, birthdays, and anniversaries provided more opportunities to be together. We attended reunions with our extended families, where sometimes our sons joined us. And, of course, camping continued to be a favorite activity as sometimes one or both sons and their families caravanned with us to enjoy the outdoors.

After serving in Ione for fourteen years, FJ left in 1994 to serve a church in Oregon. For the next twelve years, he pastored churches in California, western and eastern Washington, and Nevada. He retired from his chaplain position in the Army Reserve in 1999, at the rank of major, and then retired completely from pastoral ministry in 2006.

FJ: Carole's storms of pain-filled episodes seem like large, drenching, pelting raindrops hitting the ground so hard they splash. These bombarding splashes become streams of pain washing through her body. Most people understand the raging impact of fierce storms. Many of the millions affected by invisible disabilities suffer debilitating pain. Some may ask, "Can someone enduring seasons of extreme bodily discomfort have days blessed with jubilant sensations, making them feel as if a gorgeous rainbow just filled the entire sky?" The answer is yes!

I've witnessed the lift of divine hope and comfort that raises and holds my wife in God's intervening care. His love penetrates the indescribable stinging aches she sometimes feels. Seeing her suffer is exceptionally hard emotionally, even though I had my emotions removed. I strongly recommend having such a procedure. Seriously, though, when people ask how I'm doing, I answer, "Hanging in there," because I feel heaven's presence and am comforted.

A rainbow with all its colors delights the eyes; our diverse activities form a rainbow of pleasant times. Vacations have offered varying opportunities to appreciate time without pressure concerning the day's schedule, activity, or location. In earlier years when the boys were still home, we visited the scenic marvels of several national parks whose scenes display awesome natural beauty. Our Yosemite days remain a standout memory. Other family vacation times included visits to Lassen Volcanic National Park with its indescribable mountain and volcanic scenes offering a feast of visual grandeur. And, of course, we visited that wilderness wonder, Yellowstone—a place to see forests, mountains, wild animals, volcanic thermal attractions, lakes, and waterfalls. What a rainbow time that was!

More rainbows and sunbreaks in our life strengthened the belief we wouldn't always be tempestuously tossed on billows of pain. The sun shone brightly when our sons graduated from high school and college. When they began a deeper spiritual walk, it brought comfort to our souls.

The joy and inner peace of mind and spirit Carole experiences during ongoing physical suffering testifies how God, the heavenly Father, puts love and faith in her. She withstands her ordeal because His great love penetrates even the most awful cloud of pain. How she maintains faith and hope to live her life is difficult to explain and hard to comprehend, apart from knowing God's love is truly that strong. I simply see it and know it is so.

Grandchildren—Yay!?

Carole: Special gifts from God: seven grandchildren. Gifts, yes! Nevertheless, enjoying these gifts proved frustrating at times. I had trouble lifting a gallon of milk, so how could I pick up these precious babies? Answer: with great difficulty.

The restless, fussy newborn granddaughter had been awake many hours, and nothing would placate her—except Granma holding her. Sighs of relief permeated the room as she nestled in my arms, growing sleepy. This pattern continued with each baby, making Granma a popular person. Their parents loved this gift of mine.

When tiny, the grandchildren posed no problem to hold;

propped against my shoulder, they were protected. But when they learned to wriggle, safety became an issue. As they grew old enough to control their heads and shoulders and understand not to make sudden moves, holding them again posed little danger. During those months in between, holding the babies securely was impossible, and I was only part of their lives from a distance.

Picking up a toddler was problematic. Babysitting them by myself was unsafe. Some things I could do. Change diapers—ugh! Hold them with support—until they wanted to move. Read to them—yay! Otherwise, this Granma, full of love and enjoyment, relegated herself to the status of onlooker while others interacted with the babies and toddlers. Nevertheless, each grandchild brought joy to our lives.

And then. Oh, joy. They matured enough to talk and play. All enjoyed reading with me, crawling into my recliner until they grew too big to fit, a highlight of my day. Some loved puzzles, and we delighted in the many hours putting them together, as my strength allowed. I enjoyed teaching them to cross-stitch and to create things with plastic canvas, and one still crafts an occasional project as an adult. We played table games as they pulled a card table close to my chair, enabling me to take part too.

As they became teens, other interests replaced Granma-time. Outings—skiing, waterslides, sightseeing—displaced games and hobbies. So many times, they went without me because I lacked sufficient strength for the trip. At other times, they adapted plans, enabling me to join the fun. It was a wistful time for this disabled Granma as I wanted to go along but knew my weakness would shorten and diminish their good time. Or if they changed plans, I felt bad for the necessity.

FJ: More special happy memories are the births of grandchildren. We were present when four were born. Naturally, every grandchild was and is totally fantastic. Our hope and prayer for them is they each find the purpose for which God created them.

Thomas Carlyle, 1795–1881, stated it well: "The man without a purpose is like a ship without a rudder—a waif, a nothing, a no man."

These are our hopes for you, dear grandchildren. We pray every one of you lives a virtuous life of useful purpose. Live your lives with the awareness of your reason for being. God, the Creator of all, said in Jeremiah 1:5, "Before I formed you in the womb I knew you." May every day you live be a celebration of a life of purpose. Grandchildren, you bring a gladness of heart to Granma and Granpa.

Respites and Flare-Ups

Carole: For fifteen years, the Silent Stalker remained quiet. But his previous damage now produced increasing weakness, residual pain, and fatigability. These years resembled a roller coaster: slow climbs for respites and quick drops for flare-ups.

Welcome sunbreaks filled respite times. A temporary lessening of problems might only last a few hours, a day, or a week. Occasionally, the letup continued for a few weeks or months. FJ and I used these breathers to enjoy activities we couldn't normally experience. Sometimes, that meant catching up on unfinished tasks. Other times, we enjoyed day trips or visited friends. We were always grateful for the breathing space of days of calm and sunshine, even though the actual weather might be cold.

Flare-ups brought boring, gray days of mist, drizzle, and showers—gloomy days of coping with all the challenges. Stormy weather, complete with gusty winds and flashing lightning, continued to surprise us.

FJ's responsibilities increased as my capabilities decreased. More and more household tasks fell to him. He became the primary driver, which involved him in all shopping trips and doctor visits. Vacations, when we should relax, instead caused more work for FJ. All these changes meant less time for his projects.

44

During this period, my "spells" increased to three a day. One doctor prescribed a medication that decreased their frequency to near zero. What a relief! Two years later, they returned. By 2005, my disabling "spells" averaged one every four days.

FJ: Johnny Cash wrote a song about a boy named Sue. Why that name? Because that name would cause Sue to get tough and survive the difficulties of life. Sometimes, I think being married to someone with several neuromuscular diseases is like being a boy named Sue: either you man up and stay with your spouse or chicken out and leave.

A person with compassionate love may feel like the king of Israel in ancient times who wrote, "Oh, that I had wings like a dove! I would fly away and be at rest" (Psalm 55:6). But love is a bond of commitment, and you do all you can. The thought of getting away from Carole's pain occasionally came to mind, but it never remained as a viable possibility longer than a few moments. Where can I fly away to find rest? For me, it is and has been worship of God. All these have encouraged me: private prayer, singing and hearing Christian music, listening to Bible-based preaching, and fellowship with other believers.

Having a bouncy attitude is crucial. The Holy Spirit gives me faith, hope, and charity, resulting in a positive attitude. Nehemiah 8:10 instructs us, "Do not be grieved, for the joy of the LORD is your strength." Jeremiah 17:14 encourages us, "Heal me, O LORD, and I will be healed; Save me and I will be saved, for You are my praise." When the spirit of bounce departs, mental and emotional gloom settle into my inner self. I use willpower. I reach outside myself to call on special people, compassionate soul-friends who always encourage. Precious, caring friends help restore my bounce, especially when we get together in spiritual fellowship.

Progressive Weakness Continues

Carole: Shopping, especially for groceries, proved challenging as my strength deteriorated even further. Riding in a motorized cart still helped but even reaching for items fatigued me. As we moved around, we lived closer to stores. Eventually, FJ had to shelve the purchases. Now, he sometimes must do the shopping by himself.

In 1994, after several months of remission, which I assumed portended complete healing, I decided to clean nine sets of mini blinds at our new house. Since I was "healed," I washed them in the bathtub. The heaviness of wet five-foot-wide blinds, combined with not stopping for rest, resulted in my third-worst back spasm injury, ending my remission. I berated myself: "How could I be so stupid?" and "Why did I think I could do just anything?" Accusingly, I thought, "Again! Why does another injury always surprise me?" Unfortunately, that wasn't my last misjudgment. Times of unexpected weakness continued to amaze me.

At a Hawaiian beach in 2001, a scary event occurred. I ventured into the edge of the gentle surf. Surprise! Unable to keep my balance, I fell. I could push up to my hands and knees, but weakness, combined with an ebbing and flowing tide, prevented me from standing. Shocked and alarmed, I looked around for help and spotted Tom and FJ nearby, playing on their boogie boards. Since neither one realized my predicament, they couldn't help me rise. I continued sitting in the surf until Tom saw me and came and helped.

Lacking the strength to get back up frightened and upset me. In his autobiography *Ghost Boy*, Martin Pistorius expressed my feelings perfectly: "Feeling so out of control was daunting. Adrenaline pumped through my body, and my powerlessness felt more overwhelming than ever before as I confronted the sea."[9]

During this period, there were always a few women in each new church who helped us with housework and extended friendship to me. What a blessing they were! Women also helped me

46

pack whenever we moved again. Men helped FJ load and unload the U-Haul. Several times, one would drive the U-Haul, towing our car, while FJ drove the pickup and another trailer. Thanks to Hazel, Frances, Nancy, Billie, Karen, Jennifer, Penney, and Judy for friendship, cleaning, and packing. Thanks also to Hal, Hank, Barry, and Wink for loading and driving.

Questions for God

Carole: By 2004, my life had become very restricted and isolated. Along the way, spiritual questions arose. I have often revisited the frequently recurring theme of why God lets this continue. Why doesn't He answer our prayers for healing? We're serving Him, so why doesn't He remove this suffering? In 2004, I journaled an answer that, for me, still applies: "It's God's choice whether I'm weak or strong; because of who He is, His answer is okay with me." I expanded this conclusion with these three thoughts.

- First, I can only say this because of who God is: a God we know loves us beyond our understanding. I concluded He would not leave me hurting and weak if any other way would serve His purposes.
- Second, if it serves His purposes, considering who He is, how can I say no? Therefore, I can only give my voluntary agreement, meaning that even if it were possible to change things, why would I, since it would mean saying "no" to Him? Easy to say; hard to mean. Without a doubt, I'd rather be whole and strong, but if God sees that letting the awfulness continue is better for an unknown-to-me reason, I have to agree.
- Third, nothing is wrong with periodically checking to see if He still feels the same. God's plans might change, and He might heal me.

FJ: So many times when Carole has experienced remission, we have rejoiced, hoping the storm of pain had finally ended. How many times do rainbows appear only to have clouds cover them? Again, Carole needs to do what this favorite hymn speaks of. "Simply trusting every day, trusting through a stormy way; even when my faith is small, trusting Jesus, that is all."[10]

Someone may ask, "If trusting Jesus is so beneficial, why doesn't He heal me?" God may answer our prayer in different ways. Sometimes, He heals. At other times, He may plan to do it later. Unfortunately, to our way of thinking, His answer may be no. As He said to Paul, "My grace is sufficient for you" (2 Corinthians 12:9). Suffering may be a witness of encouragement to another person. Finally, God may stay quiet; those times test our faith but strengthen us in the end.

Sometimes, we focus our attention on wonderful-looking things we desperately want. Through hindsight, we realize our lives are better because we didn't receive what seemed so desirable. Carole's healing is something I dream about and hope for, but for now, I accept a no, praising God her condition isn't even more pain-filled and devastating.

2005–Present

Silent Stalker Reappears
Carole: As if he needed to rectify his neglect, in 2005, the Silent Stalker reentered my life with increased fury. As unstable and unpredictable as our life had been for twenty-five years, we had become accustomed to it. We didn't expect the drastic changes ahead. The Stalker unleashed storms unlike any we had seen. Clouds burst, dropping their rain when new problems appeared. As weakness and pain increased, lightning flashed, and thunder roared. Winds gusted and whirled while we attempted to accept these serious changes. Thankfully, they didn't all happen

simultaneously. We even had a few sunbreaks, albeit fewer than before. With more storms come more opportunities for rainbows. We enjoyed those days to the fullest.

Post-polio syndrome was diagnosed in 1984, explaining some problems. Years later, we finally received diagnoses which revealed the causes for more of my difficulties. In 2005, the movement-disorders neurologist diagnosed dystonia, specifically cervical dystonia and writer's dystonia. And in 2009, my primary care doctor, confirmed by a rheumatologist, diagnosed Sjögren's syndrome. Looking back at my life, I recognized conditions that had been with me, in a milder form, since childhood. I could see how the disorders had progressed.

When dystonia was diagnosed, it was a huge breakthrough. This rare disorder causes unwanted, involuntary movements, which the individual can't stop. Cervical dystonia affects neck and shoulder muscles which results in bobbing movements or in pulling to the side. Writer's dystonia affects fingers and hands, producing involuntary movements and dexterity issues. Sjögren's syndrome is an autoimmune disorder primarily causing dryness—dry eyes, dry mouth, dry skin—but it can spread to any organ. In my case, it also caused neurological issues.

Later, in 2012, my second neurologist diagnosed generalized dystonia affecting muscles anywhere in the body, creating unusual, twisted posture and movements. These cause my ribs to easily become misaligned, causing abdominal pain. He also diagnosed paroxysmal nonkinesigenic dystonia (PNKD), a rare form of dystonia. PNKD partially explained the "spells," which had again exploded with almost daily occurrences.

Botox, the most common treatment for dystonia, is a neurotoxin that paralyzes the specific muscles injected. The doctor must figure out which muscles are malfunctioning, decide how much Botox to use, and inject the correct muscle. If put into the wrong muscle, it causes weakness, lasting a few weeks. The effects of Botox are temporary, requiring repeat injections. For me, it has a twelve-week cycle, taking effect in week one or two, reaching full strength around week six, and wearing off about week ten. Botox improves my quality of life; it reduces pain, helps me hold up my head, and relieves the pulling. Polio-caused weakness precludes receiving Botox in my hand; otherwise, I'd end up with a non-functioning hand. My thoughts about beginning Botox were, "If people can use it to look good, I can use it to regain my life."

These three—post-polio syndrome, dystonia, and Sjögren's—together with their interactions, caused the unusual symptoms that had confounded so many. Doctors believe a synergy between these three major diseases caused symptoms not specific to any of them.

Before 2005, if I deemed an activity important, I could usually adapt and compensate and do it with enough planning and time. But that all changed! My ability to function became unpredictable. Sometimes, strength was available, but increasingly it was not—no matter how badly I wished or even needed to do something.

FJ: Whirlwinds of physical changes caused our life to suddenly veer in strange directions. The year 2005 saw Carole's life again wildly impacted by neurological torture. Our sons and I were once again witnessing our Carole grow weaker and suffer mutating pains. On and on, we observed her continual pain; it was a whirlwind of hurt inside her.

I remember a ceaseless parade of strange physical challenges. I saw her body react in indescribable ways. Driving on a curvy road in a blinding blizzard on a dark night characterizes trying to predict oncoming physical responses to never-ending changes. These years were increasingly perplexing. It was one day at a time, trust in the Lord, and hope and pray without ceasing. Sometimes the unremitting discomfort would cease for part of a day and occasionally several days. How did we endure the heartbreak of more physical debilitation? Hope in the Father Creator has sustained us, and we know ultimately heaven awaits us where there is no crying or pain. But we continue hoping God will yet give those golden years we heard of when younger.

Changes and New Problems

Carole: The weakness, now explained, continued to worsen. More functional ability disappeared. Swallowing problems intensified. Laryngospasms increased in frequency and severity. Lung muscle ability declined. Co-morbidities caused a decrease in mental acuity; I sometimes forgot words, family and friends' names, and how to do easy, familiar tasks. My storms produced new problems: gastroparesis, Raynaud's disease, neurogenic bladder, and small fiber neuropathy. (Reminder: check the glossary for unfamiliar terms.)

Unrelated problems complicated our lives too. Just as for anyone else, age-related changes occurred, exacerbating existing problems. Enter arthritis and other orthopedic conditions. My gallbladder quit functioning in 2006, requiring surgery, which brought on severe back spasms. In 2007, doctors discovered a cerebral aneurysm. The ophthalmologist diagnosed glaucoma in 2012.

Intermittent swallowing problems—oropharyngeal dysphagia—while not disabling, has proved a significant frustration. Envision how many times you swallow during a meal. Think about the discouragement of having difficulty swallowing even a few bites during most meals. Now, imagine a diagnostic test that involves swallowing food or liquid, but the entire test examines only four to six swallows. How lucky you must be to catch the problem when it only occurs intermittently! Catch it they did, finally. The modified barium swallow showed the cause of initiating and completing a swallow was neurological. Some foods are a no-no: popcorn, unpeeled apples, bananas, bacon, most soups, hot drinks, and most lettuce. Other foods are maybes. All foods

51

require alertness when eating. This is just one more thing that needs careful watching.

FJ: This caregiver life isn't what I'd have signed up for. I would have taken health and wealth to the max along with a spiritual life equal to the Reverend Billy Graham's, whom I greatly admired and totally respected. The caregiver of a physically disabled loved one does many necessary things for that spouse. I say spouse because it's my assignment at this stage of life. The most aggravating things happen when I'm tired and have just sat down after completing the expected tasks. Another need arises, and I must pop up to meet it.

One hot summer day, I mowed our large lawn, then finished adding more siding to the shed. Exhausted, I sat down to rest. Carole, fatigued from her activities, recuperated in her recliner, trying to recover strength. Then she realized she forgot—again— to fill her water bottle. "Honey, can you fill my water?" If she attempts to get up, I know it will take even longer for her to recover. So, I disregard my fatigue and lovingly take care of her need, the humble saint I am. To know me is to love me.

I call these things pop-ups because I must get up and take care of it now. Loving someone and making their life more positive represents the good side of being a caregiver. Caregiving without monetary compensation is a life of giving love. In Acts 20:35, Jesus said, "It is more blessed to give than to receive." One vital aspect of caregiving is emotional support for the disabled loved one; there must be a compassionate concern because you care.

Lifestyle Adjustments

Carole: What happens when the caregiver needs care? FJ developed his own invisible chronic diseases: diabetes and arthritis. From 2012 to 2015, he required five major surgeries—four on his back and a knee replacement. Each, especially the back fusion, incapacitated him for weeks or months. With help from friends and grace from God, we survived, and FJ is now doing well. Altogether, these trials added to the stresses of our already stormy lives. But God is faithful, and He provided strength to endure and enjoy life anyway.

However, sometimes I thought, "No! Here we go again! Another doctor appointment, and tomorrow I see the physical therapist. Next week, FJ sees his surgeon. Can we go to town for something else? Shopping is lots more fun!"

Not only did I see five doctors, need Botox injections every three months, and have multiple physical therapy visits, but FJ also had his appointments, physical therapy, and surgeries. Overall, it seemed as if we spent much of our time seeing medical personnel.

After FJ's retirement from the pastorate, he worked a secular part-time job until 2012 when he retired for medical reasons. That created more changes for us. I loved having him around all day. We had more time for talking, going places, and just enjoying each other's company. He had more time to help me. FJ's study is attached to our garage. It's complete with a treadmill and DVD player where he often retreats to think, write, and exercise. He named it *Zion*, his place to recharge spiritually. However, he has missed the stimulating relationships he had while working.

Coming Next

If you are having trouble keeping up with everything that has happened to Carole, welcome to the club! Have a peek at what our life looks like now.

Chapter 5

Damage Assessment—What Life Looks Like Now

"[A 1942 tornado in Oklahoma] selectively ripped off only one of the wheels of a car. But the tornado wasn't so kind to the house next to the car; the entire four-room frame house was completely blown away, leaving only the front porch and a small wooden bench that had been leaning against the house."

—Randy Cerveny,
Freaks of the Storm

Carole sat in her wheelchair, glimpsing the Pacific Ocean through gnarled, windswept trees, wishing she could join her family walking to the trail's end. On that warm summer day in 2014, they visited Cape Flattery, the United States' northwesternmost tip. FJ, Tom, and Bill pushed her wheelchair as far along the trail as it would go; sometimes, the grandchildren helped. Now she sat and waited for their return. At least, she could see a tiny sliver of the ocean, and she would love the photos they would take. Meanwhile, she enjoyed contemplating nature: pines and spruces, some with burls, others bent by winds; spreading ferns and mosses indicating high amounts of moisture; and a diversity of rock shapes. Maybe the most fascinating sights were people's reactions upon seeing a woman sitting alone in a wheelchair a half mile down the trail.

That morning had presented FJ and Carole with several choices. She could have stayed at the campsite, conserving her limited energy and missing most of the day with her family as they enjoyed sightseeing and hiking. Alternatively, Carole could have stayed in the car at the trailhead and missed this time with everyone and passed up seeing inspiring scenery. Her decision to be with her family worked out well. Their life now consists of many such options.

As tornadoes leave strange damage, so do storms in the lives of the invisibly disabled. After each storm, the situation must be reevaluated. Is there any damage? Is it permanent or temporary? Is it something the individual or his family can manage? Does it need professional intervention? We assessed the silent and unseen damage to Carole and our family as we navigated our many storms. Some losses were only temporary; others were permanent. Our family could handle some challenges while others called for help from medical professionals.

FJ Adjusts

The Silent Stalker who entered Carole's life so long ago continued launching assault after assault, resulting in neurological damage to her body. Harm done by the Silent Stalker, now identified as movement disorders, has caused ongoing pain and weakness. Limitations have resulted in loss of ability to manage activities she once easily and naturally accomplished.

Changes over Time

In the past, Carole loved sewing, spending many hours making clothes and household items. When our sons were young, she enjoyed making them matching shirts. One Easter, she tailored dress slacks, vests, and shirts for both boys. She made blouses, skirts, and dresses for herself. Twice, she sewed sports jackets for me, and for a few years, they were the only dress coats I owned. In our financially lean early years, her sewing contributed to our economic well-being. The onset of her challenges considerably diminished her ability to sew. On the positive side, she still loves sewing on a limited basis. In my office window hang special curtains she designed and sewed. She knows my love of nature scenes, so she chose material depicting wild ducks flying above a beautiful wetland scene.

Sometimes, her lack of strength to attend church, to visit friends, or to attend social events has caused loneliness. For her, these periods of loneliness don't last long; after all, she has me. What more could a wife need? This may be only a little humor, but humor is a gift enabled by God that helps keep away sadness and depression.

Quick mental comprehension enables her to enjoy various intellectual pursuits. One of her favorite pastimes involves figuring out mysteries in books or on television series like *Murder She Wrote*, *Diagnosis Murder*, *Perry Mason,* and *Matlock*. Watching these episodes became more pleasurable when our children bought a large-screen television for our birthdays and wedding anniversary. In all humility, I have to say such great kids must have truly great parents.

Going out for a movie and dinner is now rare because of weaknesses affecting her ability to sit. We were pleasantly surprised recently when we went to a cinema and watched a whole movie. We had chauffeured our fifteen-year-old granddaughter to join her friends to see the updated *Jungle Book*. Imagine our surprise and dilemma when they were refused entry without an adult chaperone. Since the theater included a bar offering any type of beverage, it didn't allow youths in without an accompanying adult to stay with them. Now what? Stay and hope Granma could endure sitting long enough, or disappoint the girls? Excellent seats, with added pillows, allowed Granma to sit comfortably for the whole movie. This was the first time we had seen a theater movie in fifteen years. For your information, I ordered a Sprite, and she enjoyed her favorite beverage of water.

Help from God

Many of Carole's days are filled with hours spent battling bouts of pain that frequently wipe out her ambition and strength to complete anything. But to combat those challenges, we daily pursue this goal with hopeful anticipation: to seek the mindset that God will fill each day with the expectation of seeing His good. On most days, we have daily devotions to connect with the powerful presence of the Divine Enabler. We reach up in prayer expectantly, anticipating the Holy Spirit's strengthening of our faith. We read the Bible because it guides us into an awareness that no matter what we encounter today, God is the same Lord who has comforted us through times of pain and poverty. He is the everlasting Father in heaven. This presence of God's love has sustained both of us through countless health-hurts. God is the One who fulfills our need for loving concern. He knows the stress we feel.

People with invisible disabilities experience a longing for others to realize they face difficulties daily. There remains a deep need for one who will be their comforter through stormy, stressful trials. The heavenly Father is the only one who truly knows the spiritual, mental, and physical struggles of life and can give genuine comfort.

Caregiver Time

Over the years, the intrusion of Carole's medical maladies gradually caused more limitations for her and resulted in my taking on some caregiver duties. Even walking in a strong wind taxes her strength, and she needs my help, or she will fall. For many years, I pushed her wheelchair anytime and anywhere she needed to walk farther than a hundred feet or stand more than five minutes. Oh! The thrill of fabric and craft stores to one whose only interest is to let her satisfy her passion for such things. Eventually, we purchased a scooter for Carole. Now, with a lift on the van, I don't have to pick up anything. She can indulge her desires and visit these fabric stores by herself while I stay in the car and read a Louis L'Amour frontier adventure.

Caregivers give up personal time and energy as they help another person. They take time to care about, with, and for the loved one as they share the struggles that have diminished the weakened person's abilities. They use energy for necessary actions the other can no longer do, such as mopping, vacuuming, and the list lengthens. Caregivers take time to understand the unique difficulties of invisibly disabled people, so they can comprehend the hard challenges the family member faces. Ecclesiastes 3:4 speaks to the changing tides of trial and triumph caregivers encounter: "A time to weep, and a time to laugh, a time to mourn, and a time to dance." Caregivers rejoice when a medical treatment mitigates the suffering or limitations. Caregivers mourn with empathy because their loved one endures further mental or physical impairment; it is a time of inward sorrow. Caregivers' lives must adapt to changes in the disabled one's circumstances.

Carole Adapts

Out of My Control

"[Her body was] in utter revolt against her will . . . It would not obey any of her commands." Thus Philip Yancey describes a woman in the final stages of ALS.[11] "Aha! That's me," I said upon reading this quote. Although my body's revolt isn't terminal, it is life-altering. Frequently, underactive muscles will not obey my commands, no matter how strongly I tell them to. Other times, the muscles become overactive, causing spasms and involuntary movements despite how badly I want them to calm down. These conditions dictate our choices and complicate planning for FJ and me and for our family and friends. Plans frequently require adjustment. Occasionally, they fall through. Sometimes, it seems a waste of time to even plan. Look what happened to our plans one year.

Summer arrived, and we were going camping again! Wait. Not so fast. Our doctor told us we must stay near hospitals. Why? The severity and frequency of laryngeal spasms meant I risked death if a severe one hit and didn't release. Our plans fell through. (P.S. The spasms ebbed again.)

Overestimating my strength leads to fatigability. I excel at such miscalculations. FJ, however, guesstimates how much I can achieve much better than I do. My need for independence—and, unfortunately, my pride—factor into my decisions to do more than I can at that time.

For instance, we're enjoying time together with a friend when FJ looks at me, thinking, "You are too tired; we need to leave." I understand what he means, but I shake my head no because I'm having fun. At other times, I need help to finish the laundry but try to do it myself anyway. And when loosening a jar lid, I just don't want to ask for help.

In each of these and many other situations, the scene unfolds this way:

> Me: "I CAN do this!"
> FJ: "You'll hurt later."
> Or maybe, "You're running out of strength."
> Or even, "You're getting too tired."

This conversation is followed by me doing it anyhow and then saying, "Uh-oh! I do need help on this little part." Or, "Uh-oh! I overdid. Now, I hurt again." Or even, "FJ was right—AGAIN!"

Avoiding the pitfall of overestimating strength involves paying attention to my fatigue levels and judging how much effort a specific undertaking needs.

Fatigability. Fatigability remains my biggest challenge, as this condition affects every aspect of our life. It increases the need for planning, complicating our ability to take part in life, and it makes for a lack of spontaneity, which can be discouraging. Tiring quickly imposes significant limits on what we can do. It limits the strength needed for social interactions. Simple ventures can become major endeavors. It seems easier to avoid even trying to do things or go places than to attempt them and end up in pain for a few days, weeks, or months.

Assistive devices help curtail the fatigue. A cane aids proper balance when walking. On bad days, I use a walker inside our house. Using a wheelchair or scooter outside our home conserves energy. I save my strength for walking where they won't go. My wheelchair's comfortable seat and adjustable legs enable me to sit longer. The scooter provides independence for me and freedom for FJ. Technically, my disabilities are no longer invisible!

The freedom of a scooter to ride! Finally! FJ's back fusion was healing. He could go shopping again. We headed into Lowe's, FJ walking and me riding my new scooter. We needed to return an item and pick up screws for a fix-it job. Inside Lowe's, we realized the article to return was still in our car. In pre-scooter days, FJ would walk back out to get it. But he couldn't walk that far yet. Wait—yay! With the scooter, I returned to the car and brought the item in while FJ waited inside Lowe's. Oh, what independence I experienced!

Controlling fatigability helps control pain. Proper rest mitigates fatigue but doesn't totally prevent it. According to my physical therapist, dystonia has stressed my body so much it has little coping ability left. So, while the cause of fatigue and effect of injuries is true, it takes much less cause to produce a severe effect.

A word about exercise: through trial and error, I learned my form of weakness doesn't respond to exercise for strengthening purposes. By 2013, I reached the point where action, even good exercise, would drain my strength. However, not moving around would mean becoming bedridden. So, every day I need to be active enough to avoid deconditioning and yet not enough to beget fatigability. Twenty minutes of daily exercise—moderate stretching and gentle strengthening—works well for me. Most people wouldn't even consider this to be exercise, but it keeps me functioning.

Dexterity. Time for fun again! I love designing computer graphics, except graphics work involves heavy use of the mouse—neither of my hands like that. My right better controls the mouse for a couple minutes. My left behaves longer but less effectively. In the past, I had used plastic canvas and embroidery, but my hands and back tired long before I finished the project. So, I changed to using the computer. My creative spirit needs an outlet. It's so much fun to design and create special cards, pictures, scrapbooks, and other projects for my friends. So, what will I do? Work on the card and hope I don't pay a heavy price? Probably.

Fine motor control problems with my right hand date back to my teen years; we now know writer's dystonia causes it. To make my fingers function correctly, I must tighten my forearm muscles. For more control, muscles higher up the arm stiffen, sometimes even into the neck and back. After a while, I can no longer even use my fingers. Pain and spasms result; my fingers curl. This trouble has worsened the last few years, creating enormous problems in tackling even simple tasks. Right-hand computer typing, using the mouse, writing checks, scrapbooking, letter writing, and crafting have become difficult to impossible. At times, fingers on my right hand curl spontaneously; other times, they move incessantly, complicating taking pills, holding a glass steady, and eating. None of the devices to aid in fine motor control help me.

Life with dystonia—and the others. Synonyms for out-of-control include disorderly, chaotic, undisciplined, disorganized—apt descriptions of how my muscles function. Dystonia, the rare neuromuscular disorder, and the new weakness of post-polio syndrome, combined with the nervous system involvement of Sjögren's syndrome, work together to bring chaos. Unpredictable dystonia generates the worst symptoms. Fatigue and stress worsen it. How much my neck bobs or pulls to the right depends on the Botox cycle's timing. The doctor injects my neck/shoulder muscles with Botox to quiet overactive muscles. How much does he use? Enough to completely quiet neck muscles, which results in poor posture from good muscles being weakened? Or just enough to calm neck muscles, ignoring nearby good muscles, leaving my neck overactive? Terrible choice.

My life veers even more out of my control whenever the doctor diagnoses a new problem or an existing difficulty worsens. Just as we think we understand how to survive and thrive, our way of living changes again. Usually, that means more restrictions in our life or more daily tasks for FJ. Confronting the fear of having more troubles in the future remains an ongoing process.

Planning—An Essential Element

My propensity for planning drives FJ, Tom, and Bill crazy. But it played an integral part in my life for decades. I consider what a task entails and break it into manageable parts, enabling me to carry out more activities. Having so much time to think while I'm resting allows me to devise numerous projects. These ideas usually involve others doing the work.

Satisfactory preparation allows us to participate more fully in life and enables me to achieve more. Even though happenings can rarely be spontaneous now, we can go see a nearby wildlife preserve, run into town, or take a "walk" with my scooter on a good day. Longer undertakings, though, such as trips, family visits, and social occasions, require pre-planning.

Even good strategies can fail because of overestimating my strength. My energy levels constitute a critical consideration in planning any endeavor. Energy conservation defines my life, forming the basis for my decisions. As one doctor put it, "You have limited strength; you can use it all at once and suffer exhaustion the remainder of the day, or you can alternate action with rest and keep going." The latter option appeals more. Sometimes, though, essential jobs use up my strength in a few hours, necessitating rest for the balance of the day. Ugh! Since energy levels fluctuate easily, estimating them ahead of time becomes a challenge.

When planning, we analyze how long the activity will take. We consider what we can do ahead of time. Locating a place to rest is crucial. Other questions need answers too. Do we need to take special equipment? Is the destination accessible for my wheelchair or scooter? Is comfortable seating available where we're heading? If eating is involved, are there foods I can swallow?

It's essential to maintain flexibility in these and other areas of our life. We need a sense of humor as we face these issues. Most important, we have to keep lines of communication open. Seeking God's guidance before planning can mitigate problems.

Pesky Dilemmas

Perplexing choices often arise. What happens when the time comes to make dinner, but I'm fatigued and desperately need rest? What should I choose when I'm exhausted but need to leave for an appointment, or want to go see a friend, or do the fun thing I had planned? I must make decisions. Should I do it and risk the damage from over-fatigued muscles? Should I cancel? Do I call on someone else to carry out my responsibility? I always tell myself I'll plan better next time. Do I????

FJ faces dilemmas as well. What do we do if his appointments conflict with mine? What happens when we've planned on attending a function and suddenly my fatigability hits? Does he go alone or stay home and miss it? What about when we prepare for a trip, and I become exhausted and unable to finish my part of the packing, yet he's tired too? How can he leave to take care of business when he isn't sure I can take care of myself?

Fatigability causes quandaries relating to social interactions. I'm limited to one hour, maybe two, of sitting up, even with a special chair. How much socializing can you do in that short time? Can you say to your friend, "I can't come in the kitchen and talk because I'm too tired"? How can you tell her the chair isn't comfortable for you? What about seminars and classes? Most last longer than my strength. Volunteering? Same problem. Using the phone? My arms quickly tire of holding it, or my voice gives out. Staying home becomes easier than venturing out, so isolation grows into a colossal problem.

Christine Miserandino, a blogger with lupus, sums up the dilemmas this way: "The difference in being sick and being healthy is having to make choices or to consciously think about things when the rest of the world doesn't have to. The healthy have the luxury of a life without choices. . . . Most people start the day with [an] unlimited amount of possibilities, and energy to do whatever they desire. . . . For the most part, they don't need to worry about the effects of their actions."[12]

Changes from Limitations

Although my limitations impact virtually every area of my life, we can adapt many tasks. By using a wheelchair or scooter, we can extend the time for shopping, sightseeing, and attending meetings. Adaptive equipment and adjustments enable me to use a computer, keep business records, do laundry, and cook with FJ's assistance. While modifications help, they have their limits; some desired activities just can't be adapted.

Using the computer avoids problems involved in handwriting. Further loss of right-hand function necessitated buying a specialized keyboard and mouse. Forming virtual relationships by the use of my first laptop (which I named "Expanded World") compensated for my limited capacity to interact on a person-to-person basis.

Loss of hand strength and function even affects cosmetic use. By choice, I only used minimal makeup as a young woman, but as I reached an age when using such aids would have been helpful, dexterity and strength losses precluded their use.

Back pain and spasms dictate my clothing styles: Will the waistband be too tight? Does it need a belt?

Foot problems determine shoe design: Do they offer enough support?

When buying a vehicle, we need to consider if it will accommodate the wheelchair or scooter.

Housecleaning has been adapted and readapted through the years. Vacuuming and sweeping were the first to be modified by sweeping, resting, then sweeping more. Over time, I quit cleaning floors. As the years passed, energy-intense jobs (deep cleaning, washing windows, cleaning bathrooms, even dusting), followed by most any housework, were severely curtailed or stopped. I can still do the movements but can't sustain them, making it unrealistic to attempt these chores. People with normal strength can carry out big or once-in-awhile jobs by staying up late or rushing through other tasks; I cannot.

Unfortunately, activities involving sitting for hours or using substantial strength can't be adapted. Alternatives include finding someone else to do it, substituting another activity, or just leaving it undone.

Family life. This storm damage affects our family too. It influences what we do on vacations, where and when we shop, what meetings we can attend together, and the outdoor adventures our family loves. It affects FJ the most.

FJ spends considerable time chauffeuring me to doctor appointments. Before he retired, having to taking time off to do so affected his employment. We must shop together as I can neither drive to nor walk into and out of stores. As to housekeeping chores, wow! We fix our own breakfasts and lunches and split cooking dinners. He does much of the cleanup. With the family's help, I still fix holiday meals. Mostly, I plan and oversee meal preparation. FJ often helps with laundry and cooking. Housecleaning falls to FJ. His involvement expanded over the years as my fatigability increased.

Our family loves outdoor activities, and we're quite pleased with how we've been able to adapt our setups to allow us to keep playing yard games, go on hikes, and experience camping trips together. What memorable times we've had. These are a few of our adaptations. I sit and rest in a lounger with a special pillow setup. The bed must be just right. We take the scooter and the wheelchair since it goes places the scooter cannot. FJ, or others, get stuck with most cooking and camp tasks. The fun we have is worth the trouble.

Most grandchildren are adults now, so they understand Granma can't do as much as everyone else. They repeatedly pitch in and help. Being unable to participate in games and fun times with them causes emotional pain and loneliness.

The unseen damage affects all levels of family life, including extended family.

Relationships beyond family. Church is an important part of my life. Although I still attend services regularly, my losses have significantly impacted my involvement. Performing church office duties—managing bulletins, newsletters, and websites—is no longer realistic. Teaching is impossible now; I don't have the strength for preparation nor breath to speak loud enough. Even extra meetings are difficult to attend; I weaken before they finish.

Friendships are difficult to maintain. Strength to go places or attend social functions with our friends often departs before the event has finished. How often do friends stick around when you have to keep saying no—or worse, cancel? Even visiting them at their homes proves problematic because of seating arrangements. Climbing a few stairs is doable but difficult. This leaves us isolated. We try to keep up relationships, but it entails a special effort.

Entertaining—in our case, having people over for meals or conversation—remains possible but challenging. I can still make special meals, but they may take several days to prepare. The key is planning: choose a simple menu or one conducive to preparing in stages, then decide on what to fix when. And FJ does any necessary housecleaning. Considering the extra effort and my strength levels, times to entertain occur only occasionally. We still love to have people over but need to limit the frequency, adding to our isolation.

Effects of Unseen Damage Everywhere
Unseen. Hidden. Invisible.

> In-vis-i-ble. adj.: impossible to see; hidden; not easily noticed.

Storm-caused structural damage to buildings often goes unrecognized from the outside; the damage is real although often unnoticeable. Likewise, damage from our life's storms often appears invisible to a casual observer. Since people cannot see anything wrong, they have trouble envisioning what I can't do or understanding why I can't undertake more activities.

My unseen damage influences what I can do at home, affects others around me, and limits social interaction. This harm alters everything in my life, but others can't discern most of the impairments.

No one is around to see me when

- I can't open a jar when fixing a meal
- I can start a job but not finish it
- Our fridge needs cleaning, but I can't do it
- FJ has to attach my <u>TENS</u> electrodes every morning and remove them every night; these electrodes deliver small electrical signals to my muscles for pain relief
- I need to choose between Facebooking with my friends or doing essential computer maintenance

Others don't understand why

- I can't play that board game with my grandkids— it hurts too much to sit
- Attending the meeting is impossible because I'm extremely weak
- I can't go shopping with them: with my limited strength I must choose between being with them or doing essential work

People don't comprehend that

- Staying up late to finish a job isn't an option; neither is hurrying around to complete the task now
- Normal chairs cause mild to severe pain lasting hours, weeks, or even months, so very specialized seating is essential
- My back muscles painfully spasm, and I risk injury if I can't lie down shortly

Friends don't realize

- When I'm standing talking to them, my legs become shaky
- If I'm weak and in pain, I still try hard to look good so as to prevent others from feeling my pain
- When I don't stand up, it may be because of my weak legs
- If I eat slowly and decline great food, I'm protecting myself from swallowing difficulties

The Toll of These Damages

These limitations have become second nature to us over the years, but acceptance—such as it is—has been hard-won. Emotionally, physical challenges are tough to accept. Everyone wants healthy and pain-free living. Spiritual questions abound. Practical issues have to be dealt with. The biggest problems may arise with relationships.

Part 2

Navigating the Storms— Living This New Life

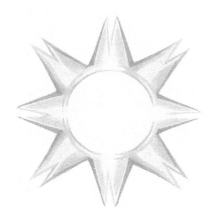

Chapter 6

Weather Disturbances Everywhere— Other Families' Stories

One July day's nationwide forecast: Red flag (high fire danger) warnings for much of the West. Flood advisories and warnings in effect in the Southwest. Heat advisories in place for the upper Midwest, while an excessive heat warning was issued for Los Angeles. A tropical storm warning exists off the mid-Atlantic coast. Quite a diversity of issues in one country on the same day.

—Carole Griffitts

One woman had lupus. A man had Parkinson's disease. Another woman was hard of hearing. A different man suffered from PTSD. This group was severely depressed, while another suffered <u>chronic fatigue syndrome</u>. And the list continued. Yet all these people looked healthy.

W*eather* is an umbrella term encompassing multiple types of atmospheric conditions. Similarly, the term *invisible disability* covers a wide range of disparate problems and impairments. They range from <u>autoimmune diseases</u> to blindness and deafness, neurological disorders, emotional illnesses, and many others. We interviewed three families concerning obstacles they face because of their invisible disabilities. Relating stories of those with difficult-to-see limitations uncovers a little-known realm where many people live. Their disabilities become their world's limiting border of life. (As a reminder, for those readers who may have skipped to this section, the words you see underlined throughout the text are included in the Glossary at the end of this book.)

Each affected person has unique challenges that involve the whole family; each story begins at varying life stages, and each family experiences different outcomes. But all share one quality: observers find it difficult to see and understand the problems they face.

Learn about these families as you read a brief background and catch a glimpse of their medical history. They contribute their ideas and experiences to the following chapters. Their input, combined with ours, illustrates how lives are affected emotionally, relationally, spiritually, and practically. Observe how they have bloomed despite their unending storms.

Jayme and Richard

It was 2006. Jayme and Richard, with their daughters—Dana, ten, and Elena, four—eagerly awaited Diego's birth in five months. Uh-oh, Jayme had the flu. At least that was what the doctor at Urgent Care, and later her obstetrician, said. Another few days passed, and Jayme visited the emergency room as her symptoms became severe. An ultrasound proved it to be her appendix. Pain meds allowed Jayme to sleep, the first time in days. Soon, she underwent an emergency appendectomy and first heard of <u>Crohn's disease</u>.

Jayme's Sunny Days

Jayme, Richard, and their girls lived busy lives. Their lifestyle echoed that of many American families. Church activities played a significant role in their lives. Dana played sports. Richard and Jayme both worked full-time.

Jayme and Richard met, dated, and married in Texas while attending college. Later, they moved to Oregon—Jayme's home state—in 2001. Travel and recreation included trips to the Pacific coast and visiting extended family in the Portland and Seattle areas.

At church, Richard and Jayme helped with youth and music; both loved creating instrumental and vocal music. Dana and Elena joined in activities with other children their ages. Jayme and Richard even participated in a mission trip to Chicago just two months before the first turbulence battered their family.

Before Diego's birth, they purchased their first home and remodeled the garage into a room for playing pool. Sometimes meals were homemade, sometimes fast food. Although the parents missed having more time with the girls, they still loved their life.

Clouds appeared along the way when digestive problems cropped up, but nothing prepared them for the tempests to come.

Jayme's Catastrophic Storm

As an older teenager, Jayme had been diagnosed with <u>irritable bowel syndrome</u> (IBS) and had suffered stomach trouble for years before the episode during her pregnancy. Her often perplexing and even unpleasant medical odyssey began then, lasting even to this day.

When removing her appendix, Jayme's surgeon saw definitive evidence of Crohn's disease and recorded it in his notes. In fact, even her appendix's size and condition indicated the presence of this illness. Amazingly, despite reading the surgeon's report, her primary care doctor still said, "Well, I don't really think that's what it is. I still think you have IBS." Jayme replied, "Crohn's makes sense. IBS doesn't." The doctor treated Jayme with a small dose of the mildest medication for the duration of her pregnancy.

Even with treatment, Jayme's condition worsened following Diego's birth. Yet, both her primary care doctor and <u>gastroenterologist</u> still only diagnosed probable Crohn's as they considered her tests "inconclusive." For the same reason, they refused to offer aggressive treatment, ignoring both the surgeon's notes and her symptoms.

Jayme returned to the job she loved, but she could only work part-time because of her physical infirmities. Despite having an understanding and generous boss, she resigned the next year, adding financial woes to the family's other stresses. Jayme's symptoms made it difficult to care for newborn Diego and her young daughters. Richard's responsibilities increased. Besides working, providing childcare, and doing housework, he had to cope with his emotions concerning a hurting young wife.

The wind and rain of severe problems troubled their family over the next several years. Jayme experienced weakness, fatigue, and multiple disagreeable digestive and bowel problems. When doctors pressed her to describe how she felt, she answered, "Like a tiger has clawed scratches through my entire bowel, and then someone has forced me to drink lemon juice."

Jayme's Continuing Storms

In 2009, their family moved back to Texas to be near Richard's family. Doctors in her new community regarded the Crohn's diagnosis seriously and treated it appropriately. She underwent surgery she might not have needed if the Oregon doctors had treated her more aggressively. While her primary doctors helped her, she still endured disbelief during several emergency room trips for pain and dehydration. Those medical personnel believed neither her history nor her pain levels, and the visits proved unproductive and frustrating.

The Texas doctors diagnosed and treated several other diseases. Although only in her early thirties, Jayme's diagnoses included rheumatoid arthritis, degenerative arthritis, fibromyalgia, and costochondritis. Disturbing symptoms accompany these illnesses. Complications of fibromyalgia include brain fog, muscle issues, and memory difficulties. Even though doctors tried various medications, the drugs often caused more problems than they solved.

Again, Jayme and Richard, with their three children, moved back to Oregon—this time near Portland. Now, she receives excellent medical care. Her current doctors have changed and reduced the number of her medications. Her challenges still remain, but her medical team wisely manages her conditions, resulting in lowered pain and improved days.

Meanwhile, family life continues. Even though Jayme's role as a mother is severely impacted, the children are growing up well-adjusted and responsible. Dana and Elena are adults; Diego is in high school. Richard still carries the heavy load of providing for the family, taking care of Jayme, and doing housework.

Jayme's entrance into Stormyland occurred gradually throughout the years; no specific date can be pinpointed. Sometimes her problems were merely weather disturbances; other times, they were downpours, and occasionally, a thunderstorm appeared—until finally, they became catastrophic. Throughout the next chapters, Richard and Jayme add thoughts about their feelings, experiences with the medical community, changes in relationships, and ideas on spiritual reactions.

Jean and Andy

Andy rushed Jean to the emergency room, bringing baby Jim and toddler Jacob along. She was suffering a severe headache and also

*experiencing dizziness, near-fainting, slurred speech, numbness, and
mild paralysis on her left side. She described the pain as a ten, on a
scale of one to ten, with an occasional thunderclap of agony thrown in.
After ruling out a stroke with a CT scan, doctors diagnosed a severe
<u>migraine</u> and admitted her to the hospital. Three days of treatment
later, with the pain level down to five, they released her. But now
what? How would Andy work? Who would care for the children?
How would housework be done? Between Andy and good friends, the
concerns were taken care of. That time.*

Jean's Sunny Days

Andy and Jean met, dated, and married, expecting a normal life.
They enjoyed their life filled with nonstop activity. Jean finished
her bachelor's degree. Both were heavily involved in volunteer
church work. Jean played the piano, organized conferences, and
did outreach activities, including coordinating and distributing
food baskets, visitation, ministry to the elderly, and evangelistic
events. Although Andy was an ordained minister, he worked at
a secular job, volunteering his time in ministering. Andy served
on church committees. He covered community events for the
pastor: offering prayer at city council meetings, helping with
the needs of non-church members, organizing outreach events.
He preached for pastors of other churches during their absences.
Andy spoke at special events such as retreats, Christian school
chapel services, youth camps, and revivals. He performed wed-
dings, funerals, and retirement ceremonies for church, community,
and military people. Andy worked full-time, and Jean worked
various jobs until Jacob came along, when they both agreed she
should stay home with him.

After Jacob's birth, Jean remained busy. She continued her
volunteer work. For fun, Jean enjoyed shopping, visiting, and
crafting with friends. She loved going out with Andy. Taking
care of two dogs and managing the household kept her even

busier. Added to all that, she taught music lessons. Being a mom to Jacob and Jim completed her active life.

Given Andy's long hours at work and church, family activities were simple: taking the boys out to eat or to a park, watching movies at home, and playing in the yard. Vacations were rare but thoroughly enjoyed.

Jean's Initial Disastrous Storm

Jean's headache began several days before the emergency room visit, growing progressively worse. When she experienced stroke symptoms, Andy and Jean realized it was time to seek help. They were relieved to find out she didn't have a stroke, but the migraine's severity upset them. Little did they know how migraines would impact their lives for years.

Jean's Stormy Life

Jean considers that her sudden entrance into Stormyland began that day in the emergency room. Even though her storms weren't life-threatening, they quickly destroyed her quality of life. Through the years, she ended up hospitalized with migraines multiple times. Her symptoms compounded to include several sub-types of migraines. These headaches can wax and wane twenty-four hours a day, seven days a week, for months at a time. Her longest migraine lasted thirteen and a half weeks!

Paula Dumas says this about migraines: "Like ice cream, migraine comes in a variety of different 'flavors,' and it 'tastes' different to each of us. Yes, the base ingredients are the same, but symptoms and severity can vary by person, attack, and over time."[13] Six weeks after the first hospitalization, Jean saw a neurologist who diagnosed a rare form of migraine. Many people have migraines, but few can imagine the anguish Jean suffers from this kind.

Seven years after her first migraine, Jean began to feel unwell again and again, experiencing many strange symptoms. In addition, she caught any virus in her vicinity. Jean had developed a compromised immune system. Diagnoses of multiple autoimmune diseases followed: fibromyalgia, lupus, chronic fatigue syndrome, and psoriatic arthritis. These diseases—and others still undiagnosed—complicate their already difficult family life.

Despite the severe limitations and pain Jean lives with daily, she still accomplishes a surprising amount. Sometimes she can do nothing; other times, she can ignore the difficulties and continue to work. Pain accompanies everything she does. Jean has one published book so far. She loves teaching piano and holds recitals for her students. She volunteers on a limited basis at her church. Occasionally, she speaks at women's conferences. Because she works hard to overlook the pain and problems, many people don't realize how much it costs her to do this.

Throughout these hardships, their family has remained a cohesive unit. The boys learned to live with their mom's limitations and became successful young adults. Andy has continued to be a loving and caring husband, supporting Jean throughout her trials. Friends helped along the way, especially in the earlier years when childcare and household help were desperately needed.

In the next few chapters, we will share Jean's and Andy's contributions of how they are prevailing in life despite stormy times.

Gary and Kathy

What a gorgeous sunny day to enjoy three-on-three baseball with church friends. As Gary played, he knew he was tiring too quickly. In addition, his chest hurt. Kathy noticed his face becoming progressively grayer. Even though Gary was eleven problem-free years post quadruple bypass surgery, they both realized he was having a heart attack. They hurried to the hospital in this small town 40 miles from their home and 125 miles from the nearest large hospital. Doctors rapidly diagnosed a heart attack, but instead of calling for the helicopter, they ordered a small fixed-wing aircraft for a faster transport to the city. That told Gary and Kathy it was an unusual heart attack.

Gary's First Cataclysmic Storm

Gary, Kathy, and their three sons lived the typical American life with jobs, school, sports, and church. About age thirty, Gary experienced symptoms of heart disease; however, every <u>EKG</u> proved inconclusive. This pattern continued for ten years, at which point additional symptoms surfaced—trouble breathing, a throat that hurt, and pain down his back. Strongly suspecting heart disease, the doctors performed a <u>stress test</u>. Three days later, Gary underwent an extraordinarily successful quintuple bypass surgery. Just four months later, he returned to work full-time.

Experiencing the symptoms, undergoing surgery, and recovering his health proved a stressful time for Gary, Kathy, and their three teenage sons. But how wonderful to have a healthy Gary back!

Gary's Sunny Interludes

Notwithstanding the severe and traumatic nature of this first storm, it did end. For the next eleven years, Gary and his family enjoyed their normal activities. The boys grew up and left home. Gary and Kathy both worked. They continued to be active in church. Times of sunshine, mixed with fog and rain, occurred.

Although lightning struck that day of the baseball game, Gary survived his heart attack. He and Cathy enjoyed seven more sunny years before the downpours returned. Even though Gary had no heart issues during those years, he developed diabetes.

Gary's Storms' Reappearance

Gary and Kathy's residence in Stormyland began after these sunny interludes. Life ushered in storm after storm. Yet God enabled them to thrive despite heavy rains and strong winds.

Gary's heart hadn't been working well, but his body had adjusted to the fatigue. He realized he could still accomplish much if he stopped and rested along the way. When doctors diagnosed congestive heart failure, it seemed like a hurricane.

Doctors put in a pacemaker, then evaluated Gary for a heart transplant. To be considered, the patient must have end-stage heart disease that won't respond to surgery or other medical intervention. These serious symptoms must be accompanied by irreversible pulmonary hypertension. Evaluators also consider other criteria.

In August of the next year—eighteen years after his bypass surgery—he had a second heart attack, a mild one. Doctors then approved Gary for a heart transplant and added him to the waiting list. Since his other organs were normal in the interim, they put in a mechanical heart to prevent a massive heart attack. Doctors operated on Gary's birthday, the tenth of September, and he returned home the thirtieth, Kathy's birthday! He returned to his part-time job as a groundskeeper.

In April of the following year, Gary received a new heart. His heart was four times the normal size; it had collapsed the lower part of his left lung. Lightning, thunder, and gusty winds from a monstrous thunderstorm struck: something was wrong with the new heart. Severe complications resulted, requiring two more surgeries. Afterward, Gary had to relearn how to walk and feed himself. He needed to regain other skills we take for granted. Two months later, he had recovered enough to go home, and by September, he returned to work again.

Gary and Kathy often wondered if Gary's smoking history, which started at age five and progressed until he became a regular smoker by high school, contributed to his problems. They also thought he might have been exposed to Agent Orange in Vietnam, where he serviced planes on an aircraft carrier.

82

Gary's Catastrophic Storms

A tsunami inundated Gary and Kathy two years later when his kidneys failed. He could no longer work because of his three-times-a-week dialysis treatment. Gary qualified for a kidney transplant because his new heart and other organs were in good shape. These stormy times proved difficult for both of them. Kathy still worked.

Yet more storms were to come. Another two years passed, and Gary developed prostate cancer. He underwent radiation even though he still required dialysis—an unpleasant combination. Meanwhile, the possibility of a kidney transplant was on hold.

Another two years passed, and doctors were ready to return him to the transplant waiting list. But peculiar symptoms emerged. He had unusual blood blisters, and a cold that began in February but wouldn't go away. Even though the doctors administered regular blood tests, they somehow missed seeing that his normal white blood cells were depleting.

On Mother's Day, Gary told Kathy he needed to go to the hospital. Kathy knew he never said that unless something serious was wrong. So, off to the hospital they went. Tests showed extremely low levels of platelets and red blood cells, resulting in a diagnosis of acute myeloid leukemia. Even with chemotherapy, his prognosis for survival remained at fifteen percent. Gary's reaction? "Well, fifteen percent is better than no chance." So, they tried it. But, six weeks later, Gary's storms ended, and he entered the forever-sunny days of heaven. Kathy and their sons' storms of grief began, but with God's help, they are prevailing even there.

Kathy adds insights regarding emotions, relationships, and spiritual observations in the following chapters.

And Even More Stories

People affected by invisible disabilities live all around us, but we often remain unaware of their problems. We know of other families living with a variety of difficulties, each with a unique story. Here are vignettes of seven other families residing in Stormyland.

Beverly is a wife and mother whose problems began after an accident as a young adult, resulting in arthritis. Adapting her work environment enabled her to continue working for years as a physical therapist. Later, she developed migraines—less serious than Jean's, but still painful and debilitating. Receiving Botox treatments for her migraines, taking proper care of the arthritis, and dropping to part-time work allowed her to continue to help her clients and take care of her family too.

Middle-aged, **Jim and Jenna** both face invisible disability challenges. Jim's painful neurological problems make his job more difficult, but he can still perform his duties. Jenna spent two years seeking a diagnosis following sudden-onset pain and weakness. Within one week, she had difficulty walking, had no strength, and could barely lift her arms. She received a referral to a rheumatologist who carried out extensive testing. Even though he couldn't reach a definitive diagnosis, he treated her with a heavy dose of steroids; these caused serious side effects. She had a nerve conduction study and a temporal biopsy that revealed nothing. But her problems remained.

Two years later, another rheumatologist (incorrectly) diagnosed rheumatoid arthritis but ignored her leg weakness. Finally, her doctor sent Jenna to a neurologist who diagnosed her problem. His conclusion: a fall two years earlier had resulted in damage, including the weakness, but it would heal itself—after two years! Since the two years had already passed, she soon returned to normal. She has healed from the steroid damage and is doing fine. Now only Jim continues to deal with challenges. Jenna's situation reminds people that some long-standing difficulties do end, and pursuing answers is critical.

Wes's service in Vietnam exposed him to Agent Orange. Decades later, he developed multiple disabling problems. Now, Wes and his wife Bonnie must rethink their retirement plans.

Medical incompetence blinded **Jerry** in his forties, changing his life forever. Along the way in his new life, his caregiver Cathy became his wife. Now they work together to make the best of his invisible disability. When you first meet Jerry, you don't notice his blindness. But you wonder why he doesn't move around normally.

Tracee, a single mom, worked full-time while raising two children and enjoying life. After thyroid surgery in 2005, she frequently experienced kinks in her neck. Suddenly, in 2016, she developed extremely tight muscles and spasms in her shoulders and neck. Her physical therapist and endocrinologist said it was cervical dystonia; a neurologist confirmed it. She educated herself about the condition and discovered there is no cure, only treatments. Tracee endures intense pain to walk, drive, and even eat as her head pulls left and down almost to her shoulder. As a single mom raising two teens, she must still work; her coworkers are supportive and helpful. She displays an upbeat attitude toward life, saying, "My family and I have chosen to live and deal with this condition in the most positive, humorous way we possibly can." Tracee overcame her dystonia symptoms with the serious procedure called DBS (deep brain stimulation) surgery.

As a forty-something, **Sam** enjoyed her career in executive management at a major bank in Australia. While on vacation with her husband, Peter, her body reacted strangely. This began her decade-long odyssey in Stormyland with an idiopathic rare bone disease and other serious chronic illnesses. Sam's bones thicken and then break, resulting in intense pain and requiring multiple surgeries. She medically retired and began a new career as a blog writer and founder of a large Facebook group dedicated to helping people cope. She also writes for other venues. Peter is her full-time caregiver.

Army Specialists **Nick and Shelby** both suffer from traumatic brain injury (TBI) and post-traumatic stress disorder (PTSD) sustained from injuries in Afghanistan. Upon returning to civilian life after their medical retirement, Shelby said, "Going back into the civilian world, people see you and think you're fine."[14]

In Conclusion

These stories represent a small sampling of conditions that cause invisible disabilities. In the following chapters, we will include input from these people and ourselves to display approaches to living with unseen hardships in four areas: practical issues, emotions, relationships, and spiritual questions. You will find how we coped—or didn't cope. From these experiences, we offer hope and tips for the dweller and understanding for the observer.

Chapter 7

Storm Consequences—Practical Responses

Water droplets combine with specks of sea salt, ash, pollen,
and dust in summer rains. Dirty raindrops cause messes.
In practical terms, those messes need cleaning.
—Carole Griffitts

Sitting in the Ione parsonage, Carole looked at her couch sporting colorful flowers on an eggshell-white background. Wait! That eggshell was now a dull, yucky tan! That couch sure needed cleaning. A few years before, she would have brought out her vacuum and upholstery cleaner and restored the eggshell color in less than an hour. Now, however, she sat there and looked at it and wondered what she could do. If she tried to clean it all at one time, she knew she would injure her arms and back again. She decided to clean one section at a time, taking several days to finish it. The couch ended up clean, and Carole didn't hurt.

As those living in Stormyland represent diverse conditions, so their practical responses will vary enormously. We share principles that can apply or be adapted in most cases, and we relate events that each of us have met in our storms.

Carole Looks Out from Within the Storms

Adapting and compensating describes our way of life. All persons with hidden limitations of necessity modify their life activities. To avoid further injury, in my case, this meant evaluating my strength, energy, and pain levels when considering any endeavor. Blind or deaf people assess their abilities realistically. Individuals with mental conditions de-stress their lives and forgo activities others consider normal. Someone waiting for an organ transplant makes major life changes. People with migraines alter their environment, darkening a room or shutting out sound.

Principles and Adaptations
Principle #1: Listen to your body. Your body tells you what you can and can't do if you listen to it. For example, a blind person can't see a dazzling sunset no matter how much he desires to. But he can develop other senses a seeing person may not. While waiting for his heart transplant, Gary could not engage in his ordinary life activities, although he desperately wanted to.

In Jean's daily life of pain from multiple sources, especially her migraines, she blends listening to her body with ignoring its messages—not always successfully. On many days, she spends the first four to five hours "sicker than a dog." Of course, that exhausts her. Naturally, Jean is then behind on her plans, so she pushes, pushes, pushes. When her problems began, she "majorly overdid it," trying to do everything she used to do. Jean learned to leave tasks undone but then felt guilty. Even now, on her good days, she runs herself ragged trying to make up for those tasks left undone.

Like Jean, I learned to do only what my strength allowed. I decided early on to listen to my body because I tired of the resulting pain from choosing to ignore it. That pain kept me from accomplishing necessary or even fun tasks. My limited strength meant catching up later wasn't an option.

Principle #2: Assess the situation. Jean asks two questions of herself: "Do I absolutely have to do this? Does it need to be done today?" In addition, she believes the husband and wife need to assess the situation. Hopefully, they can agree on how the needs can be fulfilled.

When yesterday's normal becomes today's impossible, changes must be made. At that point, realistically determine what you can still do. Maybe a change of perspective will help. Sometimes, your standards will change. Perhaps the tasks may have to be left undone, or you may need to hire someone. Ultimately, accepting your life has forever changed and finding new purpose may be your best choice.

Principle #3: Use your strengths. Vital steps to a successful life involve evaluating our personalities and recognizing our positive attributes. Determining our strengths helps make the most of our remaining abilities. This enables us to mitigate our limitations.

When I look back at my healthy and strong life, I see strengths that now enable me to make more productive use of my uptime. I had always been a planner and organizer. Now, I evaluate, prioritize, and, most importantly, segment. First, I evaluate—not always successfully—whether I am still capable of carrying out the task. Then I prioritize the array of activities clamoring for my attention. After that, I cut the jobs into smaller parts. Once in a while, I put aside high-priority tasks to complete less urgent jobs. Thus, I use my downtime for planning and organizing, and when my strength returns and I get up, I'm ready to work.

Principle #4: Accept help. All of us must learn to accept—and even ask for—help. Admitting we can't do something can be difficult, especially when we've been independent people. Acknowledging our limitations is vital to living successfully in storms. Accepting help is an essential skill to acquire. For me, I had to let others clean our house. In Ione, women from our church performed routine housework and spring cleaning.

One time, we traveled to the Portland airport to pick up our soon-to-be daughter-in-law from Thailand. While we were gone, the men in our church repaired the parsonage, and the women cleaned it for the upcoming wedding. Upon our return, we found a sparkling clean house. Our friends had spruced it up from floor to ceiling! Our appreciation knew no bounds. Those people have our eternal gratitude. May God bless them for their compassion.

Principle #5: Move forward. An arduous challenge involves accepting the changes in your life, letting go of the past, and looking forward to what comes next. This principle can be difficult and painful to implement, but it's essential for positive mental health. To move forward with your physical challenges, you need to consider practical issues. These responses will depend on your specific circumstances.

Finances

A change in financial circumstances remains a common occurrence for many Stormyland dwellers.

Some dwellers, like Jayme with her Crohn's, had to quit work. That halved their family income. In Jayme and Richard's case, they chose to live with relatives for many years, which worked well for their family. For other people, that may be an unworkable disaster.

Others, like Gary, received disability pay because of his heart issues, lowering their family's income.

Even before Jean's severe problems began, she and Andy had decided she would stay home with their boys. So, in their case, family finances weren't affected. She teaches a few piano students for extra income.

In early 1980, we dreamed of the time after FJ's graduation. As improvement continued, following my second back injury, we believed a return to strength was approaching. We expected a church to call FJ as pastor, and we looked forward to our new life and to me being a stay-at-home wife and mother. Since FJ's calling was to pastor in small rural churches, we assumed I could work part-time and still spend time with our sons. However, I was never able to return to work. Neither did I qualify for disability. But God cared for us; He provided for necessities and even a few extras.

Medical bills comprise a common source of increased expenses for most people living with invisible disabilities. Some families continue to have excellent insurance, but others lose theirs. Medicare covers people with disabilities, but it can leave bills unpaid.

Another cause of increased expenses is the need to pay to replace lost services. The outdoor person may no longer be able to shovel snow or mow a lawn. There may be a need to pay for housecleaning or childcare. Vehicle repairs may have to be done by a professional.

Time

How do dwellers fill their time? They used to work, volunteer, play sports, or enjoy hobbies. For some, when abilities diminish, an abundance of free time results. For others, a time squeeze results. Now what?

Gary kept up with his normal daily life—or at least a lighter version—for several years, but his later need for dialysis forced big adjustments. Those changes resulted in many empty hours. Gary watched television. When able, he visited patients in the hospital.

I read, study the Bible, and plan activities for myself and others.

Jean found a new career: writing inspirational books.

Sam Moss writes for her own blog and one called *The Mighty*, records a podcast, and administers a sixteen-hundred-plus-member Facebook group.

Still others find new hobbies they can do from their chair or bed; some even make money from these pastimes.

Each dweller needs to use creativity to find a workable solution.

Daily Life

Jean struggles daily with incredible pain. How does she accomplish so much? She says, "I just have to ignore the pain and push through. It's extremely difficult. I mask what is really happening for a variety of reasons. God carries me because I cannot carry myself." That approach works for Jean but not for everyone. You must accurately judge what you can and can't do.

You may need to adapt your environment. In our case, two areas required changes. First, I spend hours reclining and reading, but holding a book is difficult because of my weak arms. Hence, I designed a system to hold the book. Second, spending time with family is important to us. So, when we lived in Ione, FJ built a special daybed for me so I could be in the living room with him and the boys. We had no money in our budget to buy one. However, Ione's lumber mill had a scrap pile where local people could scavenge for pieces. FJ discovered many pieces for sundry projects, the daybed being one.

Recreation Moments

Family time may require changes too. Hiking has been part of our family's life since the boys grew up enough to walk longer distances. When Bill was four and Tom seven, we began taking mile-long walks in our neighborhood, progressing to hikes of up to five miles.

We began serious hiking in 1978 after my first injury. Over the years, my ability to hike three to five miles with relative ease declined to the point I could not stroll even a hundred yards unaided. We began using a wheelchair, but that became a problem with FJ's serious back issues. So, I now do "hiking" on my scooter with FJ walking beside me. If poor trail conditions preclude taking the scooter and FJ's back is feeling reasonably well, we use the wheelchair.

Camping differs now too. We started with a tent, graduated to a camper, and changed to a nineteen-foot trailer as my challenges increased. Even trailer life must be adapted. Sleeping in a trailer bed requires customization. Equipment must be modified for my needs. In 2016, we bought a generator to charge my scooter and electrical devices. But we still camped, sometimes with our sons and their families.

Again, imagination is the key.

Plans for the Future

More than most people, those living in Stormyland must consider their future, especially when they have a progressive condition. What further adaptations and help might we need in days to come? Might assisted care or home modifications be required? Will downsizing be necessary? Have possible financial changes been considered? If the spouse or caregiver becomes incapacitated or passes away, what will happen? What if that person needs surgery?

Looking ahead and making plans can avoid pitfalls. Andy and Jean spend time proactively considering and discussing possible arrangements. That might sound morbid to you, but these necessary talks can be constructive.

When purchasing our home a decade ago, we faced a major remodel. At that time, I weakened and fatigued easily but only needed a wheelchair outside the house. However, since we didn't know our future, we widened the doorways—just in case. Our foresight paid off; now, when I use my walker, there is room to maneuver.

FJ Sees the Storms, Inside and Out

Mobility Aids

Aging with limitations brings increased difficulties. For those encumbered with disabilities, crowded rooms and restaurants, stairs, and inaccessible restrooms impede participation in activities. The need for mobility aids adds a troublesome dimension to a family's lifestyle. An important practical issue is extending the dwellers' ability to interact outside the home.

Life gets complicated when a wheelchair is needed. Carole needs it to extend her strength whenever she leaves the house; thankfully, she can still walk around inside our home and for short distances outdoors.

A caregiver needs the physical ability to pick up the wheelchair, push it around, load it into the vehicle, and lift it back out again. Wheelchairs vary from lightweight to heavy-duty; they need to be chosen according to the needs of the disabled one. Ours weighs thirty pounds, but lifting it entails some awkward maneuvering. When I was younger, our car was a fun, snappy Chevy Celebrity Eurosport. To put the wheelchair in the trunk, I picked it up, swung it over, and laid it flat. To take it out, I had to bend over and pick it up, an awkward movement that was hard on my back. When we needed to replace our Chevy at 225,000 miles, we bought a used Pontiac Transport van, and loading and unloading became less of a back strain. To hoist the chair up and forward to push it in required less physical exertion on my back muscles and spine.

My advice is to buy the vehicle easiest for the caregiver and the one being cared for. Since the days of loading and pushing a wheelchair, I've had four spinal surgeries. I'm thankful for my past strength to manage taking my wife on walks, pushing her in the chair. I'm still grateful for the marvelous places we visited because she had a wheelchair.

At last, the time arrived when we could buy an electric scooter and accompanying scooter lift for the Chevy Uplander van we owned by that point. Since she drives the scooter onto the lift, there is no work for me. She can independently shop or sightsee. At home, a four-wheeled walker enables Carole to move around without me pushing a wheelchair or walking alongside to steady her. A cane suffices on days when she's stronger yet still needs help to maintain her balance. She enjoys these devices that enhance her personal independence. I, too, appreciate these mobility aids because, as one can imagine, I'm freed to accomplish other things.

Intervals of Relief

When we lived in Ione, respite times of togetherness that brought joy flowing into our spirits came as we read books while Carole rested on the daybed I made for her. One book we read together was Frank Peretti's thriller *Piercing the Darkness;* unfortunately, neither of us remembers the story, since that was back in the eighties. We enjoyed reading George MacDonald's dramas set in Scotland in the 1800s. If we ever finish writing this book, we intend to read more books of mutual interest again. Reading is just one way we've enriched our relationship.

Another delight we share is sky-watching. Clouds resemble pictures in the sky, and the variety of blues intrigues us. Carole enjoys seeing clouds change shape as they scoot across the windy sky. Sunrises and sunsets amaze us with their varied colors. Gold at times, purple-pink-tinged clouds, even an occasional green. Dawn and dusk exhibit a delightful panorama of hues. We share the joy of creation together, observing flowers magnificently decorated with their many colors. The array of tints and hues produce a scene beyond imagination. Animals, trees, flowers, sky, clouds, lakes, rivers, sea, and mountains entrance us and lift our spirits in thanks to the Maker of all things.

Safety Issues

One important area of practical necessities is providing safety for physically challenged people in the home. Grab bars in bathrooms need proper installation and placement for support while climbing in and out of the tub or shower and provide aid while bathing. Another grab bar should be reachable for balance issues while getting on and off the toilet. All grab bars should be securely mounted to the wall.

Preventing falls needs thoughtful consideration. A walker for getting around in the house is necessary when the disabled person experiences occasional instability or dizziness; problems with weakness may dictate a need for full-time use. Nonslip rugs help keep loved ones upright instead of having to take them to a doctor because they fell and suffered a broken bone. Different invisible disabilities necessitate consideration of other safety issues.

How alarming when the caregiver hears an unexpected cry for help from the person they care for. One morning I heard a desperate cry for help from the bathroom. I rushed there and found Carole had fallen, fully clothed, into the tub. She lay at an odd angle, preventing her from getting out. I suggested if she could turn over to her hands and knees, then grab my hand, she could climb out. Why did this happen? She sat on the side of the tub, leaning over to pull up the stopper. Her slick pants, poor balance, and awkward stretch led to the unexpected fall. This accident could happen to anyone, but who would have even dreamed of such a combination of circumstances? The point is to be as careful as you can because unexpected conditions occur in unusual ways. When thoughtful safety aids might have prevented the hurtful incident, the caregiver undergoes distress.

Because a disabled person sometimes can't get out of their place of rest, such as a special chair, a phone should always be within easy reach. If the need for help is immediate and operating a phone is something the person can't do, a medical device with a call-for-help button is useful. Carole uses a smartphone and can contact me on my dumb phone if I'm outside, in the garage, or out on an errand. Though, of course, the most advantageous aid for the disabled person is an on-the-premises caregiver alert to circumstances suddenly requiring help.

Medical Matters

Surgery and illnesses can hinder us caregivers from helping our disabled charges. We may be temporarily unable to perform our obligations to the disabled person. Necessary surgeries affected my ability to care for Carole. After recovery, though, I could provide better care.

In the earlier days of Carole's disabilities, I endured two hernia surgeries in four years. Later, within a three-year time frame, I survived the following surgeries: neck fusion, C5-6; back <u>laminectomy</u>, L3-4 and 4-5; knee replacement; back <u>discectomy</u>, L4-5; and back fusion, L3-4 and 4-5. Each surgery disabled me for weeks to months, leaving me unable to keep up with Carole's care. I was unable to do many of my normal tasks: Feeding Tahoe, our dog. Taking Carole grocery shopping. Assisting during her "spells." Helping periodically with meal preparation, laundry, doing dishes, making the bed, vacuuming. Doing yard work. Performing trivial matters that popped up.

For months after my surgeries, handling the wheelchair and pushing her were beyond my physical ability. Sometimes, one of our sons or a friend provided transportation for Carole to go grocery shopping. At church, men lifted her wheelchair from the vehicle and pushed her up the ramp into the worship center. In addition, they placed a chair for me next to Carole, enabling my back to heal.

Carole had fewer surgeries than I. Amidst her limited-functioning years, she underwent carpal tunnel surgery on both wrists as well as gallbladder surgery. On a practical level, these times increased the level of care she needed. They meant more trips to doctors, more pain for Carole, and less ability to function. When these medical trials were combined with the added impact of ongoing neurological diseases, her suffering was a tangled web of pain.

Throughout our storms, I have seen doctors, nurses, physical therapists, and technicians who understand their patients' needs.

Dedication to study and training prepared many medical professionals to administer the best treatment. As they bring relief, the patient jubilantly says, like Clint Eastwood, "Go ahead. Make my day."

When a medical provider cares enough to discern the impairment and impact of a life change on the patient's physical ability, it's wonderfully uplifting. The patient may communicate gratitude by using this song's title: "You Light Up My Life." Such appreciation frees the disabled to feel better, enabling them to accomplish more tasks related to their life needs, thus decreasing their caregivers' work.

Laughter

Humor may not seem like a practical issue, but an ability to laugh relieves stress for the caregiver and the one needing care. It's a pleasing alternative to complaining. Amusing observations don't deny the difficult circumstance; rather, it connects the person to other people.

Humor comes in various forms, from the dark and macabre to the gentle, kind, and unsarcastic. Jeffrey Boyd, a psychiatrist treating chronically ill people, says this about humor:

> It has healing properties. It defuses tense situations and allows folks to be more human, offering an invitation: *Look, let's step outside this situation and see how absurd it is.* Because sickness is so grim, others often treat sick people grimly. Laughter can turn the grim to a grimace and then into real glee. Often humor rescues human sympathy and respect from the jaws of tragedy.[15]

Carole's gallbladder removal proved unsuccessful since she still has too much gall. Carole knows I'm kidding, so she told me to

98

leave these words in. (I thought she would want them deleted. But that is her way, so often appreciating my efforts to make her laugh. After all, for me, she's the best woman on the planet, so I want her to experience the fun of whimsy.)

Caregiver's Life

Added responsibilities. As Jayme's Crohn's and other conditions worsened, Richard's responsibilities increased, even though he worked full-time. Housework and laundry became his job. With a baby and two young girls, childcare needs fell more and more on Richard. He said, "You do it yourself, or nobody does it." He believes his childhood was a great preparation time as his mom had taught her boys to cook and do housework.

Andy's life experiences paralleled Richard's. Their sons were still preschoolers when Jean's migraines began, and Andy likewise worked full-time. They had to work out plans for their boys' care, the housework, and care for Jean too. Friends helped, but friends have busy lives and can only do so much.

The first two years of our storms were intense, and my responsibilities were heavy. I worked part-time while studying for my master's degree. Household chores and childcare duties fell to me. When I graduated and became a pastor and Carole no longer worked, my workload eased. She could do light housework and laundry. She cooked juicy, tasty meals; even now, the memory makes my mouth water. She helped the boys when needed. Through the decades, as her abilities declined, my workload increased again.

As in the beginning, I now frequently clean house, cook meals, do dishes, and wash laundry. Even though I'm retired, yardwork and vehicle maintenance remain my responsibilities. If we had more income, we could pay to have more of these tasks done. My health has declined, and we're fortunate to have a part-time housecleaner helper who does so much. One good thing is Carole maintains the ability to take care of our finances—which is a blessing since I resist doing math.

Healthy living. One physical therapist says, "Motion is lotion." Another declares, "Use it or lose it." A third one asserts, "Use what you have." Exercise is critical for any caregiver's well-being. We lead such busy lives it may be hard to find time to do it, but if we don't take care of ourselves, who will take care of our loved ones? A word of caution: avoid over- or under-exercising. If you need guidance, see a physical therapist your doctor recommends.

Diet is another facet of self-care. Remember what your mom or dietitian said and eat healthy. Take the time to prepare nutritious meals for yourself and your loved one. This can be expensive, so identify resources you can use.

Proper medical care for yourself is important in maintaining a healthy lifestyle. Have regular checkups and follow any recommendations.

Balance time needed for caregiving with time for yourself.

For healthy emotions, everyone (caregiver and limited one alike) should practice a focus adjustment. Look for positive aspects in life and dwell on those to the greatest extent possible.

A Final Word

Many chronic illness problems result in disability for millions of people. Part of life has been taken from them, and there is a time of shock resulting in personal grief over their loss and pain. What would these people like to hear when well-meaning friends and acquaintances greet them? During the time of grief after his wife died, many people expressed sympathy to Ron Hall, but many of these sayings worsened his anguish. He observed, "There were just a couple of people who did know what to say: 'I can't even imagine how you must be feeling, but I just want you to know that I love you.' Those were the people who climbed down with me into the pit of my grief and stayed with me. But the grief pit is a pretty nasty, slimy place, and most people don't want to get down into the pit with me."[16] These sayings can easily apply to the invisibly disabled and their caregivers. They have lost the ability to enjoy normal life activities. So, on a practical level, be aware your words can impact others in unexpected ways, both positively and negatively.

Chapter 8

Turbulent Weather Impact—The Collision of Emotions

"The sky was dark and gloomy, the air was damp and raw, the streets were wet and sloppy. The smoke hung sluggishly above the chimney-tops as if it lacked the courage to rise, and the rain came slowly and doggedly down, as if it had not even the spirit to pour."
—Charles Dickens, *The Pickwick Papers*

The mother stared at the photo from the past with tears in her eyes, mute from her emotions. Her four-year-old daughter held a broom, taller than herself, sweeping the floor. She was the mother; that should have been her job. Why should her daughter have had to sweep?

Strong emotions assault everyone occasionally. But persons living with invisible disabilities face additional stresses. Negative and difficult feelings overwhelm them at unexpected times. Such is the case of the mother watching her child carry out what should be her duties. People newly diagnosed or undergoing unidentified losses experience perplexity and bewilderment. They can be especially prone to powerful emotional upheavals.

As the dweller, Carole feels and works through an array of emotions, but as the observer and caregiver, FJ must resolve his emotions. Jean and Andy, Jayme and Richard, and Kathy add their insights too.

Carole Feels the Storms

During my first two stormy years, frustration dominated my emotions because I couldn't carry out what I considered my responsibilities while processing a life of severe pain. Later, as it became clear the limitations and pain—thankfully, more moderate—would be lifelong, other emotions surfaced.

Positive Emotions
Even though dwellers often experience negative, or even destructive, emotions, we also know positive, happy times—our rainbow days. There is hope for the future, and even for now, as we trust God. Joy can happen any time—a beautiful sunrise, an unexpected visit from a friend, or a happy book. Love exists even during ongoing stormy times. Peace comes without warning as we experience a time of respite. Patience is a quality we learn in our awfulness. Giving or receiving kindness encourages us. The faithfulness of a spouse or friend enriches our life. Gentleness is a special treat others give us.

Negative Emotions
Fear and worry. These two emotions can be interchangeable, or one may cause the other. My longest-lasting emotion has been fear, not of what I faced at the time but of what the future might hold. These fears have often caused worry, and worry about questions in my life sometimes turned to fear. Would my

"spells" paralyze me one day? How about my pain and weakness? Will I be able to accomplish the tasks I need to? How much worse will things get? What will my future look like? Following FJ's three minor strokes, I had to consider the possibility of life without FJ. What would that be like? When a new pain surfaces or the normal pain exacerbates, it can consume my thoughts. Will it happen again? Is it an additional problem? Or an <u>exacerbation</u>?

Jean also faces these fears. When another migraine occurs, she wonders how long it will last. Her lupus flares again, and she thinks: "How bad?" She catches another virus, and she asks, "What now?" Jean copes with the fears and worries by seeking God and His presence.

In 2011, I asked myself, "Will I lose my ability to walk?" My legs had been weakening for several decades, but by that point they were declining even faster. I approached these uncertainties by remembering God had helped me in the past, so I could continue to trust Him for assistance. Next, I recalled my exceptional family's help and support and knew practical problems could be solved. I talked to my neurologist for his view. Finally, I recognized the daunting prospect of facing another loss, having dealt with so many in the previous five years.

The most important way I cope with apprehension now is to remember Psalm 34:4. "I sought the LORD, and He answered me, and delivered me from all my fears." Max Lucado says, "Feed your fears, and your faith will starve. Feed your faith, and your fears will."[17] Looking to Jesus is the best antidote for fear.

What other ways can you approach and overcome your fears? First, identify and name them. Look for the actual cause. Ask yourself if there is a sound reason that fear might come true. If so, plan a strategy. Find out more information from your doctor. Process your alternatives. Join a support group. If necessary, accept the unpalatable but don't give up hope. If you find no valid reason for fear, seek the source of the angst, and assess your feelings and the reason for them.

Frustration and anger. Dwellers' challenges frequently overwhelm them. Jean has reached a point where she realized she couldn't take on one more thing; now, how could she do her work? Then one more thing would happen, and God's grace got her through. Life hasn't been what she imagined; her plans remain unachieved. Countless days are just too much: she can't grocery shop, cook meals, take trips, or even walk across the street. Few days are satisfactory. She can't remember "normal" anymore.

Jean's concerns resonate with me. They're so familiar. Overwhelmed emotions lead to frustration, which results in unpleasant reactions. In my case, I get peevish. Too often, FJ is the recipient, requiring him to exercise extra restraint not to react. It's unfair for me to boil over at him when he wasn't even aware of the reasons. I need to remember what I once said to God: "Since You are the Lord Almighty, yet still cognizant of individuals, who am I to get frustrated when events don't go as planned?"

What events frustrate me? Interruptions to my plans. Poor time choices necessitating rest when I should be up. Loss of a complete day to unforeseen flare-ups. One problem gets better, but another gets worse. Trying to stand up from my recliner but needing several tries. The need to adapt as conditions change. Inability to make concrete plans for myself or others. The trade-off of a fun time shopping versus doing necessary tasks.

Despite limitations in my daily exercise schedule, I manage from time to time to build up to a decent number of repetitions (for me). Then, bang! Another severe flare: no repetitions, plus pain. More frustration.

Unresolved frustrations lead to anger. But anger can result in fear, worry, and depression. Any of these can contribute to frustration. Now, an unpleasant cycle results. It becomes imperative to break that repetition. To overcome anger, manage the other emotions. Seek help if necessary. Reading books, talking to trusted friends, checking out reputable websites, or seeing a counselor are good options.

Depression, death, and suicide. And then there is depression. Sadly, too many Stormyland dwellers face this condition. Sometimes, a sufferer needs help from a counselor or doctor. Other times, the person can overcome the condition with assistance from a trusted friend. Occasionally, a dweller can weather it alone. Defeating that emotion is critical because unresolved depression can lead to thoughts of death and even suicide.

Clinical depression has never been a problem for me, although I struggle now and then with the blahs. I often struggle to find motivation for work. But, I'm prone to mild depression whenever a new symptom occurs, or an old one worsens.

Kathy reports Gary struggled with depression at times. His biggest issue involved what he assumed people thought of him. When he was no longer able to join in their activities because of his heart troubles, did they understand or did they just consider him lazy? Another matter concerned his feelings of uselessness. Gary's losses forced him into disability, so Kathy had to work, increasing his sense of unproductiveness.

Another problem arose when friends wanted to help. When their natural desire to protect Gary from overdoing kept him from doing what he could still do, he became frustrated. But Kathy reasoned, "So what? Let him go overboard. Let him be happy." On the positive side, he understood he influenced others going through similar problems; many accepted Jesus because of his testimony. That was supremely important to him.

When I occasionally contemplate death, it isn't so much from a desire to be in heaven—or even a wish to die—as it is being tired of all the challenges. But, I sometimes considered thinking about suicide. I realized, though, continuing to think like that could someday lead to seriously considering it. Without God, I believe I would have attempted suicide a long time ago. In my early forties, even with God's help, it was hard to face a future of never being strong and pain-free again.

I believe considering death is a common reaction for people undergoing severe challenges. It seems an easy, harmless way out of problems. Although suicide controls when death happens, excellent reasons exist to choose life. The pain and guilt around a loved one's suicide may cause family and friends to be overwhelmed. Family left behind may need financial support. But consider the most important reason: life itself is meaningful, no matter how hard it may be.

People can combat suicidal thoughts in several ways: Acknowledge their remaining strengths. Find ways to make life more interesting. Realize the intrinsic value of life. Consider medication; it may be necessary if brain chemistry has changed. If you have been considering suicide, please talk to someone you trust or call 1-800-273-8255. Your life is a gift; please don't end it.

Losses, sadness, and grief.

> Sometimes loss does its damage instantly, as if it were a flood resulting from a broken dam that releases a great torrent of water, sweeping away everything in its path. Sometimes loss does its damage gradually, as if it were a flood resulting from unceasing rain that causes rivers and lakes to swell until they spill over their banks, engulfing, saturating, and destroying whatever the water touches. In either case, catastrophic loss leaves the landscape of one's life forever changed.[18]

My first back injury belongs in the instant category of loss; it caused major disruption to our lives for two years. Then gradual loss occurred when the disabilities stretched out, slowly increasing over the years, producing significant disturbances to our lifestyle. Gary's losses, too, were a mixture of the two, sometimes a torrent, other times incremental increases in severity. Jayme's disease developed over years. The first change in Jean's life occurred dramatically, while other challenges occurred over time.

To accept sadness due to losses can be challenging; sorrow may creep up on you unaware. Then you may have to reacquire the positive endurance you developed. Once, when we visited Tom's family, they had Thai relatives who wanted to sightsee. I could go on short jaunts with them, but since my weak body demanded rest, longer day trips were beyond my ability. So, I sat at home while my children, grandchildren, and their visitors toured museums, enjoyed shopping, and visited points of natural beauty. Heartbreaking for me. I'm not alone in these feelings. Many people in my Facebook groups express similar experiences.

Besides dealing with other emotions—fear, frustration, sadness, identity issues—you may have to work through grief, which is a five-stage process. First, come denial and isolation, followed by anger, bargaining, depression, and finally acceptance. View these stages flexibly, as people may travel these in a different order; individuals may skip a step or get stuck in one; steps may be revisited.

Over the years, I've grieved again and again. New losses meant a need to acknowledge and accept even more limitations. Grief is an integral part of acceptance. Sometimes, though, I wondered if I ever fully grieved and accepted or if I just did the minimum to survive and thrive.

Trusted friends and family can encourage dwellers as they face the sadness and grief of loss. Isolation only increases these emotions, so the presence of others serves as an antidote. In addition, counseling or a support group can be helpful.

Isolation, loneliness, and social skills. "As friends and family stayed away—some because they found my undiagnosed illness frightening, others because they were unsure how to comfort. . . . Whatever their reason, people kept their distance as they hugged their healthy children close to them in silent gratitude, and my family became more and more isolated."[19] Thus Martin Pistorius, the "Ghost Boy," describes his family's increasing separation from others because of his profoundly disabling condition. His observations apply to many invisibly disabled people, even though his circumstances markedly differ. FJ and I believe similar reasons apply to our growing isolation. Being cut off from friends begets loneliness. Aloneness and the reality of disabilities lead to a loss of social skills. Social interactions take energy, an element often lacking in the disabled. These problems also apply to the family caregiver.

Isolation, loneliness, and loss of social skills become a vicious cycle, one which I've been unsuccessful in breaking. How can I do better? Intentionally connecting with friends—old and new—makes a good starting place. I can use email and social media for this. I can practice cures for loneliness: focus on others, listen carefully when they talk, and remember and follow up on their concerns. This can be difficult to do amid our pain, but practicing connection enriches our lives.

Pride and self-importance. Too high an opinion of one's importance indicates a negative form of pride. Self-respect and self-esteem reflect a good sense of pride; it's proper to take pleasure or satisfaction in a job well done. This section will speak of a person being overly aware of himself.

My inability to sit for long periods has caused me several embarrassing situations. When visiting FJ during his hospitalization, I asked his nurses for a cot so I could stay near him and still rest. Often, when visiting friends, I have requested pillows so I could lay on their couch and recover my strength. Once when flying by myself, exhaustion hit during the layover, but the only place to recoup was on the terminal floor. I spotted an out-of-the-way corner, lay on the floor, and ignored passers-by. The remedy for this negative pride is to take care of my needs and ignore what others think. Maybe even laugh at my plight.

People typically take pride in their looks and appearances, but my looks suffered when I began wearing a <u>TENS unit</u>. The pain relief unit clips to my waistband and creates a bulge under my blouse. Its wires connect electrodes on my back to the unit and, unfortunately, its long wires are visible below my blouse. What a tacky look—certainly not fashionable. It limits my clothes choices to dresses with a belt, or pants, or skirts. But, oh, the pain relief!

Self-centeredness due to overwhelming life events is a special temptation for dwellers, including me. It can take over my life. Thinking only of myself causes me to ignore people and lose my ability to love others. The antidote is deliberately considering others. Start by choosing one small task to please someone else, then choose another person to encourage.

Lack of self-control is a subtle facet of self-importance. Who I am and what I want becomes of the most importance. One man put it this way: "I admit to you I am finite. I like to believe I am infinite and can control life and run my world, but the truth is I can't."[20] My biggest lack of self-control is eating. Putting food in my mouth is one function over which I have complete power. For years, such an attitude contributed to overeating. Since I have no control over so many areas, I subconsciously exercise the ability to choose, even though it hurts me. To develop self-discipline, learn effective strategies, and put them into practice, an accountability partner helps.

Changes and Coping

My personality has never handled unexpected change well. Therefore, coping with new diagnoses is difficult. When another part of my body refuses to work correctly, questions plague me. "How much more can I withstand? How many more things can go wrong? Not again," I protest. Then comes the frustrating companion thought, "Here I am, AGAIN!" More questions follow. "Did I truly think it wouldn't happen again? Why am I surprised? What do I do now?"

This last question begins the coping process. The bewilderment and emotional impact of these changes determine where to start. For me, I might read over my to-do list and then consider if it is important to carry out whatever activity I should be doing, even if I don't feel like it. Or should I substitute something constructive? Or is it better to rest? Next comes facing my current emotions. Am I depressed? What are the actual issues involved? Are there negative emotions I should resist? Am I remembering happiness is a choice, even when choosing it is challenging? What an excellent time to read my journal of good memories.

When the changes are monumental and peace is difficult to find, I return to my relationship with God. I picture a huge hand, gentle and safe. Even extremely weak and fatigued, I can still crawl up and over into this place of safety and rest. For the time being, I sense protection and can relax in the safety of God's care. When I cope with the changes, I return to my world refreshed and ready to meet more challenges.

Humor
Although not strictly an emotion, this quality enriches our lives, enabling us to thrive during our storms. "Like a welcome summer rain, humor may suddenly cleanse and cool the earth, the air and you."[21]

We can use humor as a defense. FJ often repeated the familiar saying he heard from his grandpa: "It's better to laugh than to cry." If hard times were to be my lot, laughing would be much more fun than crying.

Amusement or comedy is also proactive, providing a release as we face rainy times. Proverbs 17:22 tells us, "A joyful heart is good medicine, but a broken spirit dries up the bones." FJ excels at humor, often lifting my spirits as we face another new diagnosis or increasing symptoms. It also cools the good old everyday variety of hot emotions.

FJ Weathers the Storms

Life has become a roller coaster of a few remissions followed by renewed weakness. Emotions again must adjust to muscle strength and endurance changes, making mental equilibrium and emotional wellness hard to maintain. How Carole accomplishes any emotional balance is by holding on to faith in God and the hope He will strengthen her daily fortitude. This strengthening, I've seen Him do and am amazed.

Carole and Joni Eareckson Tada, the popular quadriplegic author and speaker, and twenty-three million others are overcomers of hard life challenges. Many persons afflicted with physical calamities, such as Carole, Jayme, Jean, and Joni, don't simply endure horrible pain and life-limiting struggles but also rise to useful, purposeful lives. As James Stewart spoke in the movie *Shenandoah*, "If you don't try, you don't do." These people are achievers despite obstacles of pain and limitations of physical activity.

Struggles and Coping
Being thankful circumstances aren't the absolute worst they could be is what helps me cope as Carole's caregiver, sharing her pain and struggles. It's possible her physical condition might deteriorate to the point of becoming immobile. As of now, she still dresses herself, so she's free from the emotional pain that comes when someone else needs to dress her. In case you haven't thought of it, that means freedom for me: one less responsibility and obligation.

113

Yet, she persists in doing everything her abilities permit while maintaining a positive view concerning the worth of her life. Her core of inner strength is why, despite incessant pain and physical weakness, she hopes her life will contribute to a better world: one in which understanding replaces a lack of sensitivity about the needs of those negatively impacted by disabled lives. Those who care with understanding for their friend or family member help produce a better world.

I find thankfulness by appreciating the abilities she still possesses to do a few chores. Every task she can still accomplish for herself—and some for me—is something I cherish. My strength is something else I'm grateful for. When the need arises to get things for her, take her to medical appointments, keep up the house and yard, make home repairs, and carry out vehicle maintenance, I'm thankful for the strength that enables me to do this work. I'm appreciative of Brenna's two hours of every other week housecleaning. When faced with a task unfamiliar to me and a sudden insight comes to mind—usually after ample time of reflection on the matter—with deep gratefulness of spirit, I offer my appreciation to the One above.

Work situations. At times, Carole has felt particularly bad and looked as though living might be near an end. While working, I experienced waves of concern for her survival, fearing she would die while I was away. It proved difficult to set aside such emotional times of worry. Seeing her so affected by her invisible disabilities upset me. When I saw her torment, I struggled with fear of the unknown. During the early phase of her unstable health and disabling problems, neither we nor even medical doctors could understand what was wrong; they saw no known reason for it. One physician said, "Her symptoms are so bizarre."

How do I handle such inner turmoil? I keep believing in God and seek strength that comes through praying, praising Him in gospel songs, reading the Bible every day, and fellowshipping

114

with other believers. My older brother often quoted Nehemiah 8:10: "The joy of the Lord is your strength." And this is true. He lifts me up in every way when I seek His aid. I still pursue His presence and help day after day because, as Psalm 23:1 says, "The Lord is my shepherd." Jesus tells us in Matthew 28:20, "I am with you always."

Fearful Circumstances

Andy experiences deep concern for the physical symptoms his soul mate endures. In earlier years, they faced the possibility of a frightening answer about the unknown source of her rare migraines. What would the children do if their mother didn't survive, and how could Andy absorb the pain of losing the woman he loved completely? Fear for himself and his family was daunting to contemplate. Andy and Jean live the storms of unending physical pain and distress, as many others do. How do families like Andy and Jean's survive and have hope for healing? Their confidence is from and by faith in the God they know loves them.

Since Jean's severe migraines' debilitating symptoms often resulted in her being bedridden, these episodes concerned Andy when he had to leave for work. He faced one fearful event while at work when Jean called and said she was having functional physical difficulties. Suddenly, he no longer heard any response from her. Their six-year-old son, Jacob, picked up the phone, saying, "Mom's on the floor and can't get up." Jacob didn't know what to do except hope Dad would come home and help Mom. Andy immediately left work without communicating with anyone. Extreme concern for Jean caused more haste than the lawful speed allowed as he raced home. He quickly drove her to the hospital, where she received emergency care. Even though they received no answers as to what and why, that episode resolved, and Jean functioned fine until the next time.

Uncertainty, Mystery, and Insecurity

After over four decades of living with a wife who often faces painful surprises, I've experienced more than my share of scares and uncertainty. She shares an abundance of information about what mystifies and perplexes her. I liken this situation to soldiers on a military patrol in enemy-occupied territory. They encounter various types of perilous ambushes and never can be certain just where the danger lies. Perhaps they could step on a land mine or be shot by a sniper; they risk injury from chemical weapons. The possibility of crippling or fatal encounters from enemy weapons causes a sense of uncertainty, keeping the soldier on edge. Likewise is the danger from the Silent Stalker during Carole's neurological flare-ups.

Patients who fight for the freedom to live without fear of physical debilitation are like soldiers fighting against ongoing ambushes. Many neurological disorders remain unidentified. Not all causes have been found. For some known ailments, no treatment has yet been discovered. Somewhat like warfare, a clear-cut answer doesn't always exist as to the dangers, hurt, and unease of many diseases and disorders. These patients may say, "Why me?" Another question plaguing the hurting person is, "How can I live with such physical uncertainty?" They observe, along with me, that after years of medical care, it continues to be a baffling, discomforting situation.

My wife and I often call this life intrusion an unending storm. Can you imagine the sensation of lightning surging like a burning fire through your body and what such pain does to a person? This idea of lightning may be exaggerated, but please think of this: Night has come, and the patient has been asleep until suddenly, awakened in early morning hours, her body begins to severely, involuntarily arch. She's tried to describe these manifestations to me, but they defy explanation. Some "arches" cause her back to curve forward, then move backward as her legs draw up toward her chest. These may last up to forty-five seconds or more. The longer these arches continue, the more severe the pain. There is good news: her neurologist prescribed a medication that helps reduce occurrences. Leg jerks, radically different than "arching," as she calls it, can occur day or night (usually night) and make up another form of discomfort; they've been with Carole for years. The words "leg jerks" are self-explanatory and are also painful and involuntary.

The mystery of neurological diseases is an ever-changing kaleidoscope of mutating physical symptoms. Patients begin to accept changes occurring in their bodies, adjust emotionally, and make lifestyle changes. Then comes the necessity of readjustment upon readjustment, causing an onslaught of insecurity. How often the sufferer longs to understand why the changes and to discern their source. Every person benefits from knowing themselves physically and figuring out coping strategies for stable living. Patients caught in a neurological maelstrom of physical adversity cherish the knowledge doctors provide. Suffering a mysterious unseen ailment creates a desperate longing in the afflicted patient to understand and be understood by family and friends.

Understanding or Lack Thereof

Sufferers with invisible physical problems are often considered lazy and sometimes thought of as hypochondriacs because they see doctors often. Multiple medical appointments indicate a search for answers and an antidote to relieve their pain. They want to know why their bodies are weak and fatigued even when attempting ordinary tasks.

Sometimes people with imperceptible diseases are shunned unintentionally by others. If the disabled person spends many hours of the day resting, acquaintances and friends might think visiting would be a hardship. Family or friends may even become tired of hearing about the mysterious affliction. The disabled person may be relating their problems in an attempt to be understood. The patient is saying, "I am still worth caring about. Send a card, phone me, or visit when I'm up to it." Who will care enough to try and understand even a little of what persons with unseen disorders endure? Why do those afflicted with invisible illnesses speak so much about their condition? Because they would enjoy being understood by people who care enough to come alongside and act as compassionate friends. Who needs a friend more than the sufferer who is often set aside?

Chapter 9

Stormy Transitions—Acceptance and New Purpose

"The best thing one can do when it's raining
is to let it rain."
—Henry Wadsworth Longfellow

Her young granddaughter wailed plaintively, "I can't go through this," as she endured the pain of the blistering burn on her fingers. Carole so identified with that emotion as she remembered feeling that way again and again. When unable to go places with her family due to exhaustion. When pain unexpectedly struck again. When she repeatedly did time-consuming personal care tasks most people do not have to. When a new symptom showed up. And on and on the list went. FJ knew that feeling too. When helpless to alleviate the suffering of the love of his life. When doing morning and night chores for Carole. When more housework became his responsibility. When driving her wherever she needed to go.

Carole Considers the Changes

Acceptance Defined

As years have passed with no improvement and more decline, acceptance has become imperative for my emotional health. As I function within the existing conditions, I search for creative ways to live with my challenges and seek new purpose for life. My family also needs to acknowledge and live with the limitations. This troublesome task of acceptance sometimes proves elusive to achieve, but we stay hopeful.

Many people who experience severe loss recognize the truth. Author Jerry Sittser, who lost three members of his family in an accident caused by a drunk driver, states, "The passage of time has mitigated the feeling of pain, panic, and chaos."[22] But when losses continue to occur, the passing of years doesn't necessarily blunt emotional pain, making acceptance harder to acquire.

We think of "acceptance" as coming to terms with something, or as a willingness to believe, or as tolerance. Applying these meanings to invisible disabilities is difficult. First, I maintain, we must *believe* our problems exist. Then we must *tolerate* these restrictions. Finally, we need to *come to terms* with them. These steps aren't a one-time experience, unfortunately; we may need to repeat these measures. Neither are these ideas easy to practice.

Although acceptance carries a positive connotation, the related word "resignation" implies a negative meaning. To be resigned involves accepting the realities of current life but with an unresisting attitude, or with a submissive mindset, or without protest. While we must accept our circumstances, we must not give up, assuming we can do nothing. At a minimum, we must have hope in the knowledge our suffering will end—in heaven, if not before.

Bill Crowder's prayer, in the devotional *Our Daily Bread*, certainly applies to acceptance. "As time drags on and answers seem faraway, teach me, Father, to find my help in You and Your presence. Enable me to endure, and empower me to trust in you."[23]

Acceptance Applied

Before 2006, I did a reasonable job of accepting my limitations. Since I realized many necessary tasks were beyond my capabilities, I either asked for help or let them go. After 2006, my medical condition rapidly deteriorated. Acceptance, but in reality resignation, meant doing only what I had to do to survive and ignoring everything else. There was no grieving because I overlooked the need to admit to myself the unlikelihood of ever regaining my strength. Because I didn't want to consider the possibility of even more limitations, I denied the likelihood of continuing losses. But even then, hopefulness lingered; heaven was in my future.

So . . . what did I do? I realized the need to come to terms with my extreme limitations. I accepted they're here to stay and might worsen. I resolved to be proactive and change my attitudes and actions to become an overcomer—to find purpose for my life despite limitations and relapses. I changed long-term project plans and scaled back my expectations. I proposed to focus on my family. I looked for ways to show compassion to others by demonstrating love, being available, making sure they know I care, praying, and following up on their concerns.

For Christians, one dimension of acceptance is spiritual. Answering the perplexing question of how a loving God can let us hurt is essential. As I mentioned in an earlier chapter, years of soul-searching led me to this conclusion: It is God's choice whether I'm weak or strong; because of who He is, His answer is okay with me. This requires ultimate trust and still is difficult to honestly mean.

In 2012, I journaled about this.

It's time to settle this question. At this point, I'm
not healed. It's God's prerogative at any time in the
future to heal me, but it's His choice. I can't bring
healing about by anything I do, not even by having
"enough faith." It's time to move on in my life. Physically, I need to get as much information as possible so I can live up to my potential. Emotionally, I
need to work on acceptance issues and leave behind
all my escapism activities. Spiritually, I need to find
God's purpose for me in my challenges. I need to
seek His vision for this stage of my life, and I ought
to search out the "good works" He prepared for me
to do (Ephesians 2:10).

I still work on these issues.

Repeatedly, though, I question the Lord, "How do I, Lord? It's
so hard. And the hard just keeps on getting harder." This stormy
life, full of terrible times, is difficult. I dislike hurting. God has
given me many gifts, but I can't use them. Life abounds with
things I wish to do. And then, of course, the big question: "You
heal others, why not me?" This is where faith comes in.

When I question again, I remember all God has allowed and
pray, "Help me accept what I can never understand—and I need
not understand. Help me disengage from the hurt of not being
healed. Cleanse me of the damage it has left. Fill me with faith
and love for You. And use me as I am." This is spiritual acceptance.

Acceptance Hindered

What makes it hard to accept our difficulties? When our unpredictable condition flares again, we wonder why. But asking why
is a useless question that upsets our level of acceptance. Flares
sometimes rob us of any positive self-worth; we need to remember

the beneficial facets of our lives. We have to realize the untruth of judging our lives worthless. When we question why we should exist or continue to exist, we deny God's plans and sovereignty. When we fall into the trap of focusing on our hard lives, we need to remember no one promised us a rose garden. Actually, I need to remember our family had twelve years of living in a rose garden. The answer lies in accepting life as it is and finding new purpose.

Self-Identity Considered

How is identity related to acceptance and new purpose? In every way.

Our sense of who we are suffers when we become chronically ill and realize it will be unending. If our identity has come from activities we can no longer do, we may wonder who we are. At least I did.

I concluded I'm more than my illness. But I wondered who I was. During the first two years, I was an invalid, barely able to leave my bed. However, I finally realized being an *in*valid—powerless to get out of bed—does not equal being in*valid*, meaning worthless. I determined to recognize the truth of this: just because I exist, I have value as a person. I had to see I am more than my problems. These understandings developed over time. I concur with this author's words: "I affirm that I am a finite physical body, and that right now I'm feeling confused and tired and a little scared. My illness has clouded my mind. My body is limited—I can't meet everyone's wishes, let alone my own ambitions and desires."[24]

We need to be careful not to confuse our roles with our identity. Before the limitations, my highest aim was to be a wife and mother, one who did wifely and motherly activities. My conception of that role expanded when I grasped that being a wife and mother was more than actions. What my husband and sons needed most was love, and I could still be loving. I just could no longer perform as I used to. It hurts very much to see FJ do most of "my" housework. And if a task, still within my ability, must be done immediately, I can choose to do it, suffer later, and watch my pain hurt FJ. Alternatively, I can delay the job if feasible, do it later, ask for help, or leave it undone.

Sam Moss, who moderates a Facebook group for sufferers of chronic illness, asked us three questions that speak to our identity and roles. First, what has chronic illness taken from you? This concerns the changes and how we view ourselves. Next, what has it taught you about yourself? Realizing who we are on a deeper level helps us in our self-identity. Last, what are the things you can still enjoy? We can create new roles for ourselves when we answer this question.[25]

New Purpose Sought

One man with dystonia found renewed purpose after he acknowledged a new sense of normal in his life. He admitted life had changed forever. He recognized and accepted humans have an amazing ability to adapt. Yet, he still needed time and the support of others to help him discover his new purpose.

How do we find ours? My search began by inventorying my past strengths and interests. Compassion and caring expressed in acts as well as thoughts formed the hallmark of who I was; the question became how I could show care now. I loved taking care of my family, extending hospitality, and working through our church. As a thirty-something woman with a husband in graduate school and young sons, I hadn't begun thinking about life's purposes.

When I could no longer ignore the unending nature of my limitations, my self-image plunged. I sought ways to find new purpose. The initial step was to accept what exists and grieve the losses. I listed activities I'd never do again: stay up all day, walk beside FJ, or teach classes at church. These activities fit my former purposes of loving my family and helping others. Were there other ways to still fulfill these purposes?

In practical terms, choosing an activity based on needs or desires rather than strength level was impossible; the usual ways of loving and helping were no longer open to me. My next steps involved realistically evaluating my current status, receiving all available medical help, dealing with spiritual and emotional implications, and grieving my losses. Then, I visualized alternative possibilities. My wish list included walking beside FJ on hikes and in stores, cleaning the house myself, doing my part when camping, driving myself, and singing again. Since these are now impossible, I must build new dreams.

For me, loving my family includes designing and creating legacy projects for our grandchildren. Visually documenting the fifty-plus years of our life has resulted in thousands of photos to choose from as I create scrapbooks, DVDs, pillows with pictures, and other family memory items.

As a couple, FJ and I envisioned fresh ideas for the future. As a couple, we started by looking to the past to see what worked, then decided if we could adapt it to current abilities. We loved both reading together and spending time in nature, but my losses meant these activities must be limited. One goal we have achieved was to buy a scooter and lift for the car; this makes fulfilling other desires easier.

Practical Aspects Adapted

Do you have a purpose which no longer works? Maybe you can modify rather than discard it. If you are responsible for your family's food preparation but can't shop, cook, and clean up in one day, you might adapt your purpose by still shopping but cooking only one meal with someone else cleaning up. Your shelves would be stocked with supplies so others could provide for themselves. In past days, my job was to plan and shop for daily dinner menus for a month. Now my goal is to plan for ten meal possibilities and buy all ingredients. In addition, I stock emergency food for those challenging days; then, either I can cook, or FJ can prepare a meal from the freezer.

Apply these steps to any purpose which no longer works.

- Examine what is involved.
- Evaluate to see if modifications are possible.
- Decide if it's outdated; discard, if so.
- Determine if it's still needed and how you can fulfill it.

We must exercise care in our evaluations. A few years ago, I realized the physical impossibility of accomplishing everything I believed God wanted me to do: run my website and blog, write this book, assist FJ in his writing, and do legacy work for our grandchildren. Then I read David Platt's book called *Radical* and realized my focus needs to be on God. Platt reminded me our greatest need is to seek God, asking Him to accomplish through us what we can't do in our strength. These thoughts gave rise to this prayer: "O Lord, You do have a purpose for my life. Even if it's only as a presence in my family members' lives. If I weren't here, they would be missing the love, prayers, and teaching that I can give." And so, I recognized God's primary purpose for me at this time is to love and be present for my family.

My Purposes Found

Four purposes emerge as important focal points in my life: praying, especially interceding for others; writing this book (and when it's finished, promoting my website); seeking ways to encourage others; and organizing legacy work. However, legacy activities are now a lower priority because of decreasing strength. Of course, other important concerns exist, such as FJ, housework, and family time. But it seems to me God has given me these four areas of significant interest on which to concentrate.

As a rule, I have lived my life and carried out my purposes with enthusiasm. Such excitement derives from God enabling me to exist, but even more, to overcome and thrive. Yet, that sense of adventure has dulled. So, I sought, and found, the problem: my purposes had become un-balanced, spending too much time on writing and too little on people. As I could see no way out at the moment, I kept trudging on. When commitments are fulfilled, I plan to focus on family, friends, and legacy work, while husbanding my strength. Writing is still ahead but I will limit my time and energy.

Acceptance and finding new purpose are easier to achieve when life is seen as a gift. Philip Yancey's quote from a cancer patient sums it up well. "I do not consider myself dying of cancer but living despite it. I do not look upon each day as another day closer to death, but as another day of life, to be appreciated and enjoyed."[26] Any invisibly disabled person can echo these thoughts.

FJ Reflects on New Life

Acceptance Questioned

New purpose? Acceptance? I am unsure about the acceptance portion of a stormy life. Ultimately, miracles still occur. So, who knows? I retain a deep-seated hope God will still make things different and give us a Godwink, a term coined by Squire Rushnell. People interpret it as "an unusual coincidence that God orchestrates." We first learned of the idea on *The 700 Club*.

We want, and continue petitioning the Father in heaven for, something we've heard called "the golden years." You know, when you live to be ninety and are strong enough to climb Mount Lassen, which is 10,457 feet high, without even being short of breath. Now, this I joyfully accept because Carole and I signed up for the golden years fifty-plus years ago, and we're still long-ing to experience that exuberance. I frequently request the Lord to bestow our hoped-for allotment of those fabled golden years. Now, this concludes my complaint concerning acceptance.

Acceptance Acquired

Okay. Here comes my statement about accepting unpleasant changes that cause adjustments and inward struggles. I recog-nize certain circumstances in life feel like unwanted stress. I find the difficulties Carole and I sometimes face in our life together to be an arduous struggle. The stress of seeing a steady loss of physical health takes an emotional toll on me. Now that she can no longer accomplish things once such an ordinary part of her life, I must make a colossal personal adjustment. She had ability in so many areas, but now these skills prove challenging or even impossible to use.

When she was younger, we rode bikes for miles at a time; now, we can no longer do that. Especially since, these days, I can't ride a bike either. My lovely young wife used to have strength enough that together we easily moved a heavy hide-a-bed couch. We washed and cleaned our vehicles every Saturday. We enjoyed drives through scenic areas. The years and neurological disorders have taken away much of her physical ability. Her balance and strength diminished, sometimes even making walking difficult for her. Mentally, she's still the brightest woman on this planet, in my opinion. She still finds much of my humor funny because she understands it, or maybe she just loves me a lot. I'm thank-ful for her ability to accomplish so much in the way of literary efforts. She, for the most part, masterminded this book. We share a spiritual bond emanating from God, causing an enduring unity and acceptance despite all the woes.

Some things have changed with the passing years. When I walk the trail near home, I'm usually alone, unable to share nature's beauty with my soul mate. So, I take our camera and show Carole pictures when I get back, letting her share in the sights of interest. There are no walks together in stores without a scooter. Rarely do we go together to a truly fun store like Home Depot or Lowe's. When we were remodeling our house, we enjoyed countless shopping trips to those stores. However, things changed, and I adapted, but I haven't become accustomed to her episodes of pain. Sometimes their occurrence makes it necessary to leave in the middle of a church service. Still, we know trying to worship with others of like faith is an important undertaking.

Purpose Modified

My purpose as a husband began over fifty years ago when I recited my wedding vows to Carole. I promised to love, honor, and cherish her in sickness and in health and in adversity and prosperity. I spoke these wedding vows as a promise to her and to the Lord God of heaven. The wedding ring is a symbol of an endless circle of loving commitment. With the strength of our Lord, I intend to keep this promise until either the rapture that takes us both to heaven or death separates us. We are His children and should treat each other with appropriate, loving respect, cherishing one another.

For the first twelve years, we enjoyed health, even though little prosperity. Then I slowly began including the role of caregiver in my purpose. As years passed, my duties increased, thus adding to my purpose as a husband. I continue to do my best to love, console, and comfort Carole as I provide the care she needs.

Chapter 10

On the Scene—Family

"We prayed. I could feel pressure, and being sucked. I put my body over them to try to protect them," Tonya Williams said about her successful efforts to save her two young children and three dogs during the 2013 tornado in Moore, Oklahoma."
—"Oklahoma Tornado Victims Astounded," Gillam/Simpson, Reuters

One sunny summer day in 2005, FJ and Carole planned a day trip to Yosemite with Tom to celebrate his visit. It was only two hours from their new home in Nevada. They stopped first at Old Big Oak Flat Road, which held memories from the boys' childhood visits when cars could drive along it to see the Tuolumne Grove of Giant Sequoias, sightseeing along the way.

Now, it was a paved, two-mile, round-trip trail. The sign said "easy travel"; it neglected to warn of the steepness. Tom and FJ traded off, guiding the wheelchair downhill, holding it back from gaining too much speed on the descent. All three enjoyed delightful scenery. One father commented to his young son, "They sure must love her to do that!"

When Carole and the guys neared the bottom, sunny skies

opened in a torrential downpour, and they sought cover under the trees. Wheelchairs. Metal legs. A thunderstorm. An unnerving thought! Tom and FJ decided to continue down and see the giant sequoia trees. After returning to Carole and waiting for the endless storm to stop, they decided to go back up, assuming the rain would soon quit. FJ and Tom pushed Carole in her chair. One ran and pushed while the other rested somewhat while running, and then they would switch places. They finally made it to their car, chilled and soaked to the skin.

Family members should care for each other even when it requires extraordinary effort. However, the demands of chronic illnesses complicate these relationships. The person experiencing disabilities is not the only one concerned. These challenges and subsequent problems affect spouses and children too. A 2008 article states, "Statistics show that over 75 percent of marriages plagued by chronic illness end in divorce."[27] One marriage expert notes, "Spousal caregivers are said to be more prone to depression than adult children who are caregivers."[28] Children may grow up dysfunctional because of a disabled parent, or the pressures may mold them into responsible, successful adults.

Jerry Sittser explains how these losses may affect family members. "Problems keep interrupting their lives, demanding more of their time and resources and draining them of energy. While they love their disabled family members, they also feel resentment, labor under constant exhaustion, worry about money, and wonder about the future."[29]

Carole Contemplates

Family

Enduring ongoing storms of physical disabilities is a family problem. While the person with the debilitating condition suffers physically, those challenges also affect the entire family. Way too late, I realized these problems are not "my" problem but "our" problem. I understand FJ and our sons hurt because I hurt, and my limitations cause extra work for our entire family—FJ, especially, and our sons, daughters-in-law, and grandchildren when we get together. I'm aware my challenges curtail fun times, such as walking together while shopping or enjoying recreation. Even understanding these truths, for years I missed the idea that my challenges are "our" problem: that they must accept my life as it is, just as I must. Each time we're together being family, it's a labor of love.

Families should not deny the realities of suffering. Acceptance involves acknowledging pain and mourning changes. Sherri Connell sums up the feelings of disabled family members like this: "After all, if they must live *with it*, we can certainly live *next to it!*"[30]

Family Issues

How does housework get done now? Someone must clean house, fix meals, and wash clothes. I had always considered these to be my responsibilities. But I know if I do it when weak, pain will follow. If delaying the task is feasible, I postpone it. If the job can't wait, either FJ does it or we pay for it. In times past, friends helped. However, FJ enjoys the challenge of seeing how much manual labor he can accomplish.

What about family income? If the wage earner can no longer work, income needs to be replaced.

When children are still at home, childcare must be provided. When Tracee's severe dystonia first occurred, her children were in

133

grade school, and her mom, Alma, picked them up from school.

Planning should be a family concern. With advance thought, we can still achieve much. But planning can have a downside too. In our case, too often, my ideas infringe on FJ's domain and mess up his plans.

Control is another problem area. Since so many things in my life are beyond my abilities, I too often want to exercise inappropriate authority over others. When FJ is driving, for example, I "need" to be sure he knows where to turn or to stop. Often, this results in me whining and FJ being upset. A false premise rears its ugly head in my life from time to time: *if I could control my world, the challenges wouldn't exist.* Wishful thinking. My problems would still be there.

We can't always decide what happens, but we can manage our attitude toward it. I try hard, frequently unsuccessfully, to incorporate that mindset into my life. When difficulties cause misery, I don't want to make those around me miserable too. The reason for the misery might be beyond my control, but the response is mine, and it affects others.

Relationship Difficulties

I whine, act peevish, or pity myself when I hurt, things don't go my way, or some task doesn't work correctly. Unfortunately, this maelstrom too often affects FJ. He supports me so well, and it's terrible to pay him back like this. Frustration causes these actions, but that is no excuse.

FJ experiences frustration, too, as he performs numerous extra duties because of me. He still has his tasks he would like to do but must stop and carry out my responsibilities. Sometimes, it overloads his day, frustrating him and disappointing me. I hurt because he hurts.

I escape my difficult life through reading. However, this positive getaway harms relationships when I read instead of relating to family members. Too often throughout the boys' teen years, I ignored them when reading, fully absorbed in my book. I still sometimes do this with FJ.

Open lines of communication enable satisfying family relationships. Jayme and Richard assert that a lack of communication can create more space between partners. Such inadequacy, unfortunately, occurs in a stormy life when family members may be stretched just doing essentials. Or the partners might be trying to shield themselves from hurt. Or it could happen because of an unknown future. Jayme and Richard wish they had included feelings in their conversations.

Communication styles differ from person to person. Kathy points out that each of her sons interacted differently, according to his personality.

Support Systems

FJ is the primary person in my support system. He acknowledges the realities of my challenges and consistently validates my worth as a person. These attitudes enable me to succeed in life. FJ never treats me as if I've chosen these challenges; he knows they are beyond my control. He always believes me when I say I'm too weak or exhausted to do something. In fact, he often recognizes the weakness or fatigue before I do. He respects me as a person.

Tom and Bill and their families make up another valuable part of my support system. As teens, they accepted me with all my weaknesses and did their best to help me. They loved me anyway. As their families expanded, each additional person accepted me. Even today, each one knows I have problems, yet they do what they can to include me in their lives.

A huge component of support is understanding. One of my first primary care doctors told me, "If your husband understands, you're lucky. If your sons understand, you are incredibly lucky. Then it doesn't matter what others say or do." I wish other people would acknowledge my problems are real and disabling. But I thank God my family understands. They form the bulk of my support system.

Tracee's teens, Eliza and Daniel, and her mom, Alma, serve as her support team. They encourage her with humor. Eliza notes they seek not to let Tracee's dystonia affect their entire lives and believes they have done an outstanding job. They accept the dystonia as something they must live with.

Marriage

Sometimes FJ must shop or attend meetings or undertake projects by himself when we would rather do it together. I experience the heartbreak of solitude when staying by myself instead of being with him; he also misses me. Thus, loneliness can invade a marriage.

We realize the divorce rate is quite high when a couple lives in the stress of unending storms. Nonetheless, divorce isn't an option for us. But when FJ watches me in scary or painful situations, it hurts him. Yet, there is no relief except what he finds in God. Over time, damaging stress can harm the caregiver-spouse. It's easy to imagine this might cause a spouse to depart. Despite the hurt and pain FJ has undergone over the years, he remains faithful and loving. And I'm so thankful for this.

Richard's friends don't understand how he could stay in his difficult circumstances, yet he never considers divorce and remains committed to Jayme, despite her battle with Crohn's and her other diagnoses. "One marriage for life" continues to be his enduring mindset.

Children and Grandchildren

Jean's Jacob and Jim are successful college students, once again proving a parent's invisible disabilities don't have to affect their children negatively. In fact, one could assert the difficulties experienced growing up strengthened them. Jayme's Dana and Elena are working their way through college. Our Tom and Bill have each been married over twenty years, are deeply devoted Christians, and have successful careers: Tom as a Coast Guard officer; and Bill as a Certified Public Accountant. Their older children are college students too.

Despite FJ's and my best efforts, the boys experienced a dysfunctional family life as teens. I couldn't accomplish the usual "motherly" things. Before my limitations, I cooked every meal and many desserts. As my disabilities increased, the quality of meals decreased, and I made fewer homemade cookies and cakes. It became more difficult for me to clean the house, so Team Griffitts—FJ, Tom, and Bill—worked to handle the chores. Unfortunately, some criticized us because we didn't require more of our sons. Because of their heavy responsibilities, we let them be teenagers whenever possible. Another consequence of weakness that bothered me was being unable to attend games and meetings with Tom and Bill. I missed so much of their school lives.

Other mothers echo experiencing these types of problems. Jean endured intense disappointment when she couldn't travel, perform activities, or attend her boys' programs. She acknowledges, though, that while her sons did fine at home, being with other children brought awareness that their mom didn't do what other moms did. Andy, however, noted kids can have fun anywhere, which his sons proved in their lives. Despite their mother's difficulties, they enjoyed life.

Tracee's Eliza and Daniel offer their insights as teens currently experiencing their mom's stormy times. Eliza speaks of the ups and downs of her mom's life. Because Tracee's muscles pull her neck so far to the left that it rests on her shoulder, she might run into things, knock down displays, or even accidentally hit Eliza when unable to see her. Eliza comments, "We laugh about all the situations it puts her in because it's hilarious." Seriously, though, she hurts when she sees Tracee in pain but can't help. Daniel, Eliza, and Tracee do their best to accept the circumstances. Eliza believes it has strengthened their family and improved their relationships. She says, "We try our best to help our mom and laugh with her when things get hard. My brother and I love our mom, which is enough for us to help her." Daniel says, "I don't know what I would do without my mom here." He speaks about her positive attitude and appreciates her desire to support others with dystonia.

Another penalty of life for the disabled arrives when grand-children do. My limitations affected interactions with our grand-children. But fun times happened anyway. Our strong love for each other overrode the complications caused by my disabilities. Even now, as teens and adults, they continue to look for ways to include me in their fun.

Parents
Parents are troubled when their child, even an adult child, faces a chronic illness. Such a strain increases when the condition affects their child's ability to function in life. Unexpected emotions surface. Sadness develops when the child finds it hard or impossible to continue working or doing hobbies. Sometimes, guilt plays a false role if the problem is hereditary or was caused by the parent's actions. Perplexity emerges if such an impairment is tough to see or challenging to understand. Disbelief can occur because the parent doesn't wish the child to suffer. When the disorder has no cure, the parent may cling to a mistaken hope that it will end.

Jayme's dad expressed his feelings about her challenges. He said it felt "really weird" she had major medical problems because he, as a parent, thought something would happen to him before it happened to his child.

Along with being sad, my own parents were accepting and supportive. I think they experienced guilt now and then because my childhood polio symptoms presented themselves on a camping trip. This was false guilt since they couldn't have known the polio virus was present.

Alma reacted in disbelief at first when a doctor diagnosed Tracee's dystonia. As with other parents, she wrestled with questions concerning why it happened and why there was no cure. She became upset and agitated because the doctors couldn't answer these questions. She even grew skeptical about Tracee's doctors. She didn't want to settle for the outcome they presented. However, Tracee helped Alma come to acceptance. Since Tracee's dystonia is severe and painful, Alma's feelings are understandable. She knows her daughter is perseverant, persistent, trustworthy, strong, and friendly. In addition, she realizes Tracee covers up her pain when possible. The sudden onset and severity of Tracee's dystonia obviously challenged Alma, as it would any parent.

FJ Considers

We asked caregivers these questions: How do you feel about this situation that changed your life? Why do you continue in this relationship? Richard answered, "I had to because of love for my spouse and promised commitment that says, 'I do, for better or for worse, in sickness and in health, till death do us part.'" Great difficulty arises from the emotional stress of repeatedly seeing the one you love in pain throughout the years. Dreams become impossible. Places to see. Vocations to pursue. Recreation activities to share. Projects needing two to accomplish. Loving fellowship from working with the one you love. Leisurely walks together in beautiful places that are no longer possible without assistive devices. Carole is no longer the person I married in terms of activities she can do.

How I Cope with Her Pain

There are times when, in moments of exasperating stress, I say to the Lord, "I can't take any more of seeing her suffer." I don't say this from a lack of love for Carole, who has endured hurt nearly every day of the past forty years, but rather, it's because sharing love with her is to share her pain. When your loved one is enduring a storm of pain, God is your hope and help. Saying *I cannot take any more* is a plea to God for her healing and hope for the future. He offers help for emotions that endure medical crisis after crisis.

Often, I feared I'd return home from work to find she had gone to be with Jesus. At times she has looked so washed out I have wondered if the end of her life was near. I have felt her body next to mine shudder in the nighttime, sometimes jerking spasmodically. Her neurological disorders cause so many bizarre symptoms. Sometimes she tries to hide the pain and discomfort, so I won't know she's going through a more-than-usual struggle.

These distressing emotions accumulate on both spouses in a marriage where one suffers and one gives care. Thankfully, we haven't come to the so-called rope's end, nor have we reached a breaking point. God has seen us through many stressful times.

"An unstable chemical that cannot be held in a neutral state" would be a description similar to how Carole's problems do not remain unchanging but erupt in new and unexpected symptoms. The unforeseen changes ambush her as they alter a health status she may have just become accustomed to emotionally. The impact of new symptoms often results in increased weakness and possibly elevated, or different, pain. The caregiver must adjust, making time for additional tasks. Living with a loved one who has multiple neurological challenges is what I call an emotional roller coaster.

Fortunately, Carole and I do more than just cope with pain and physical limitations in our marriage. We share a love that comes from God. What kind of love? The kind that brings forgiveness and confession back and forth between us. I may say to her, "I'm sorry you made me snap at you. I would never do that if you hadn't made me!" Of course, she knows I'm teasing her. She's so smart she sees my humor even if no one else recognizes it.

In addition, a daily time of reading a devotional book, singing hymns and choruses, and ending with morning prayer strengthens us. The fellowship of worshiping with friends and acquaintances encourages us. Corporate worship in a Bible-preaching, Bible-teaching church lifts us spiritually and is part of our relationship with God. We delight in being together and sharing family life with children and grandchildren, especially when vacationing together or visiting in one another's homes.

Marriage Pluses and Minuses

Marriage partners can cope with and conquer storms of adversity that sweep into their lives if they possess the pluses. Teachers put plus or minus marks for emphasis on pupils' grades. Couples in marriages with more pluses than minuses are nurturing a relationship that conquers whatever destructive forces may move against them. Both husband and wife must learn how to defeat damaging pressures that tear marriages apart.

Selfishness is, in my opinion, the leading cause of fracturing the bonds of marriage. Selfishness puts your personal desires above the other person's wishes. To overcome being selfish, I must ask and answer some questions. First, what are my wife's real needs? And how am I doing in meeting them?

One Sunday morning, Carole and I were listening to the late Adrian Rogers preaching about marriage. He told husbands they should be mindful of how they treat their wives because God is her heavenly Father, and that makes her God's girl. Who is foolish enough to mess with God's kids? This also applies to how wives treat God's male kids. Loving respect for each other is a plus mark of a marriage that endures even during severe times that seem to pull people apart.

This woman God brought into my life over fifty years ago is an extraordinarily strong person. She has strength enough to laugh in times of physical hardship. Not all the time, but more than you might think likely. I would like to share just a brief example of her reaching for humor even when she hurts.

One day she came through the living room door, home from physical therapy. Quickly, she sank down into her recliner, worn out from her treatment. I sat down in my recliner next to her, waiting to hear the therapist's analysis concerning the latest problem, severe heel pain, diagnosed as plantar fasciitis. "Well," I said, "what is that?" Carole answered, "In my case, it's an adjustment my brain makes to compensate for an incorrect manner of walking, resulting in stretching and tearing of the fascia." My layman's interpretation: it results from the brain improperly compensating for the way her foot functions. She continued, "My therapist said it's a mechanical problem rather than a neurological one."

I jokingly told Carole, "Well, honey, if it's mechanical, then I can get some tools and fix it." She good-naturedly responded with a little snicker to reward my attempt at humor. I am sensitive and concerned about her suffering, and I do try to avoid becoming callous toward it. Yet, finding bits of humor is one of the pluses that help us cope with her suffering. You may not be Jack Benny, Red Skelton, or George Burns, but a smile, a laugh, and a lot of love from the Father above is crucial.

Emphasizing the pluses as often as you can helps maintain a positive view. Being aware and concerned about how your spouse is feeling shows loving concern. Knowing and demonstrating understanding of the other's condition reveals love and enables joy amid suffering.

For me, taking on tasks I see she can no longer do and helping her finish jobs she starts but runs out of strength to complete requires knowing her limits. Not jumping in and doing everything for her involves sensing when she can finish or if her stamina is close to ending. Concern and being lovingly attentive empowers me to know when to assist and when to leave her to do what she reasonably can. Helping too much is no help at all because she will lose her diminishing personal independence more quickly. She certainly is most fortunate to have me as a husband because I can read her like a book, and I'm real humble about taking care of honey bun. To my spouse, the best I may do for her good is to show love in action by what I say and do.

Carole read somewhere that many married people desert the marriage if their spouse becomes permanently ill. In these cases of desertion, running away is an act of pure selfishness. What brought them together was likely only lustful infatuation. But such marriages can mature into relationships built on true, heart-felt, abiding love. For a description of genuine love that overcomes the stormy adversities marriages face, 1 Corinthians 13 tells it best; it's worthy of contemplation.

Spiritual Help in Marriage

Coping has no magic wand to wave over the hurting and pain caregivers see assailing their loved one. Both the caregiver and the one they care for desperately need to find a soul-healing balm, especially if the illness is long-term, permanently degenerative, or terminal. Discovering the source of that soul-healing balm may be, for some, nearly impossible.

I compare the search for a soothing answer for the perplexing angst to a life lived by an old desert rat seeking gold, silver, or other precious metal in a desolate, harsh region. The land is barren and seemingly devoid of anything valuable. The prospector learns by experience and study. He listens to others who have mastered the signs indicating where treasure is likely to be found. Upon discovering the location of these valuable treasures, the miner begins the labor of digging. Each day he digs. Imagine how he feels as the sun rises and, instead of lying about getting tanned, he must dig and dig beneath the ground all day long. Obviously, if the gold is to be his, he must toil for it.

Finding soul-healing balm is the same, except the mining is done mentally and spiritually. Spiritual mining for that healing balm is a continual process and can be accomplished by prayer and daily Bible reading. We find considerable encouragement through devotional books like *Streams in the Desert, Our Daily Bread*, and *Open Windows*.

Beware, for there is a serpent in your rose garden who seeks ways of tearing apart these precious values and practices of mutual respect and love. That serpent's bite is a potent poison. Jesus is the only cure that overcomes the serpent's venom. Selfishness and anger are especially wounding actions in the stormy world.

Carole's disorders themselves and our reactions combined have at times caused temporary distance between us that had to be overcome. Those times have felt like a hot stove I would seek to avoid. Yet God draws us together despite the hurt. Remembering experiences shared over past years helps to renew an appreciation of the trials a man and woman must fight together to have an enduring marriage.

Love between a man and woman can be rekindled if it should grow weak. Jesus said, "Apart from Me you can do nothing" (John 15:5). Our marriage of fifty-plus years endures because of the Lord's presence. Almost every day, we pray together and separately. Jesus said to go into your closet—meaning a private place—and be alone with just you and God. We make this a regular practice and find redirection when a course correction is needed. Living in a rose garden requires honest self-work that brings a beautiful, hard-won reward: a marriage with loving companionship. To speak frankly, it ain't easy. In my opinion, the harder the fight, the greater the victory.

Normal couples don't like living in a mess. A rose garden is uninviting when it isn't kept free of weeds. Carole and I work together, dream together, and plan together in a life shared happily in spiritual unity. Marriage is only as good as the couple makes it with divine help. Using the personal pronoun, I—as in, admitting *I was wrong* and asking for forgiveness—is difficult but necessary. Improve personally to avoid becoming stale and closed to reassessment as circumstances change.

Chapter 11

Responders—Medical Community

"A first responder is a person with specialized training who is among the first to arrive and provide assistance at the scene of an emergency, such as an accident, natural disaster, or terrorism."

—"First Responder," Wikipedia

Jayme summed up her advice concerning medical care this way: "No matter what the doctor says, pay attention to your body and how you know you feel. After the visit, look stuff up, investigate for yourself, and see if what they're saying makes sense."

When people initially enter Stormyland, they need first responders. They require an assessment and diagnosis of their ills, if possible. After residing there a while, though, their needs change. They must develop ongoing relationships with various medical professionals. Since these involve continuing connections, we drop the word "first" and call the medical community "responders."

Medical Personnel

The medical community is a diverse group. Interactions with doctors, physician assistants, technicians, and therapists—physical, occupational, and speech—taught us these professionals can range from knowledgeable and experienced to dangerously uninformed. Often, people with invisible disabilities, especially those with multiple unusual conditions, experience challenges in obtaining good medical care.

Most medical personnel are kind-hearted, compassionate, and caring. Thankfully, many doctors display knowledge and exhibit compassion; these professionals listen proactively. Fortunate are you to find such a doctor, therapist, or technician. When one comes our way, we don't want to change! Unfortunately, some physicians jump in to help without listening to you. Others assume they already know everything. Some disbelieve the patient. A few expect they can easily find answers for which others spent years searching. A negligible minority even act as if they are gods bestowing their perfect knowledge on you.

Healthcare professionals are taught that common things are seen commonly, but that rare diagnoses do exist. Furthermore, students learn if a more common condition fits the patient's symptom profile, it's probably the right diagnosis. Since this isn't always correct, how do medical professionals know when they are dealing with a rare diagnosis? Dr. Thomas Woodward, in the 1940s, coined the term "zebra" for us with rare diagnoses or undiagnosable problems. He told his medical students, "When you hear hoofbeats, think of horses, not zebras."[31] Thus, doctors are conditioned to think in terms of the most probable cause. For us zebras, finding a doctor open to looking for zebras can be problematic.

The best medical practitioner is one who presumes the patient tells the truth. Carole related strange symptoms to a physician's assistant, remarking, "You probably think I'm crazy." The PA replied, "My philosophy is to believe whatever my patient tells me, even if it's strange, until and unless the patient gives me a reason not to."

Egregious Examples from Carole's Experience

During Carole's first visit with a pulmonologist, he reiterated, "I SAID you don't have a breathing problem at all!" When she responded with a question about her specific condition, the doctor walked off in a huff because he assumed she was questioning his conclusion.

Years later, a highly recommended neurologist admonished her, "You don't have post-polio syndrome because I don't believe there is any such thing." Immediately following that statement, he qualified his explanation by adding there might be a few such cases, but it could only happen to those whom polio seriously incapacitated. We thought, *Honestly? You disagree with common medical thinking, but you are right, and all the others are wrong. And then you qualify your opinion!*

Along the way, a <u>physiatrist</u> (PMR), speaking of Carole's weaknesses, said, "Look around you at anyone your age. You'll see they're just like you." Later, while lunching with our son, she pondered the doctor's words and cried. But she went home, observed her friends and neighbors, and saw no one experiencing similar problems. She didn't return to that doctor.

And then there was the physical therapist. "You can straighten and pull your shoulders back because that requires less strength than hunching." Experience had taught Carole the fallacy of his statement, yet he refused to listen. Years afterward, we learned cervical dystonia did make it harder for her to sit up straight. There was a valid reason for her inability.

Rather than reacting to these situations in disgust or anger, it is healthier to laugh! Fortunately, most of our experiences with medical people have been with knowledgeable, experienced, and compassionate types.

149

Ventures in the Medical Realm

Unfortunately, Jayme's early interactions with the medical community were often negative because of the multiple doctors who denied the possibility she had Crohn's disease. One time, frustrated when the doctor wouldn't listen to her, she told him, "Just listen to what I'm telling you, and draw your conclusions from that." Jayme advises that communication between your primary care doctor and your specialists is critical. Each doctor needs to be aware of the care others give. She believes many doctors want to make an easy diagnosis rather than to accept something unusual.

Most doctors haven't treated Jean well. What does she want now? To be finished with seeing doctors. As her health became more complicated, her relationships with doctors deteriorated. Ten years ago, Jean's physician's assistant believed her and conducted appropriate testing. Unfortunately, that PA has since retired, and many other experiences have been quite negative. Jean estimates 75 percent of her doctors have offered varying excuses for not believing her. Some told her she was just making up her symptoms. Other doctors claimed she was depressed. Several insisted it was impossible to have so many things wrong. A few asserted she just did not fit the box. The nicer doctors said they didn't know how to help her, or it was probably just her autoimmune stuff.

One doctor told her he could do nothing to help unless she took the prescriptions he recommended. Jean is extremely careful about taking new medications as any drug can have side effects ranging from nuisance to life-interrupting to severe. Complications can arise when taking multiple prescriptions as they can interact badly with each other and can themselves cause new symptoms. When Jean had her annual checkup with this doctor, he didn't even do blood work. The clincher came with his declaration, "If you get bad and need some help, come back and see me." This last saying is one many of my invisibly disabled friends have heard from doctors at one time or another.

Know Yourself

The most important aspect of obtaining medical care is to advocate for yourself courteously yet firmly. You know your body best. When what your doctor says doesn't make sense to you, there are several options. First, ask for clarification. If that doesn't work, talk to others with similar problems. Do research, research, and more research. Kate Mitchell, in her blog, *Kate the (Almost) Great*, says, "Most importantly, make sure you're looking at a reputable source and, ideally, that it has recent information."[32] Then, if you still disagree with your physician, you may need to look for a new one. Kate adds, "At the end of the day, you are the one in charge. You are the patient, the one the entire appointment is about."[33]

Remember Jenna, who experienced sudden, severe pain in her legs? She pursued multiple consultations with doctors, rheumatologists, and neurologists as she persisted in seeking to address all her symptoms and kept questioning the doctors about her weakness. They kept ignoring her. As one specialist finally discovered, the cause stemmed from an earlier injury. Jenna's experience illustrates the importance of knowing your body and continuing to pursue answers.

An active young wife and mother who worked as an aerobics instructor began experiencing periods of severe weakness. She visited her doctor, who diagnosed panic attacks and wrote her a prescription. She knew herself and knew it was not panic attacks, so she stood, tore up the prescription, and left his office. After visiting a specialist, she received the correct diagnosis of hypoglycemia. Without proper treatment, this condition could have killed her if she had continued heavy exercising.

Kate Mitchell summarizes another experience by saying, "I spent several years in which doctors told me my ankle was fine, but it turned out to be super messed up. Learning first-hand at seventeen that doctors can be wrong (like, *really* wrong) has meant that I listen to and believe my body above what doctors tell me about it."[34]

So, again we say, know yourself. Stand up for yourself.

Time for New Practitioners

What do you do when you must find a new practitioner? It depends on the circumstances.

If you have been receiving incompetent care and have exhausted every avenue where you live, you might need to consider relocating. This was an issue for us when we lived in an isolated area and Carole couldn't find adequate medical care. Even traveling as far as 120 miles, it was impossible to find competent doctors and specialists who would also accept her as a patient. We moved—a drastic step indeed—twelve hundred miles back to Spokane, Washington, where we had formerly lived because we had received excellent care there. When Jayme's family relocated, her medical care for her Crohn's diagnosis improved dramatically because of her new state's quality practitioners.

When you have received disappointing care from your family doctor, think about looking for a new one. First, consult your insurance carrier because that might limit your choices. Check out possibilities with your family, friends, or support group. Look up the new provider on the internet, but remember ratings are often left by someone who strongly likes or dislikes the doctor. Consider the doctor's location and how often you need to visit.

If your problem is finding a specialist, talk with your primary care physician. Relate your concerns and ask for a new referral.

Finding help when you are new to a community can be challenging. Ask your previous doctor if he knows someone in the new area. Talk to your insurance company. Check the internet. If you know people in the new area, ask them. Find a support group and consult the members. Again, consider travel time. And remember what you need from your new medical practitioner.

New-Doctor Anxiety

Carole's ideal medical team starts with a great family practice doctor who will oversee and coordinate her care, who will be a caring listener, and who can keep track of all her problems and specialists. This doctor knows whether the current symptom is related to an existing condition or if it's new. This team's makeup continues with knowledgeable, caring specialists. This optimal situation includes an outstanding neurologist skilled in administering Botox injections for muscle spasms. At present, her team is excellent.

Appointments with new doctors, though, remain a stressful time for Carole. Numerous occasions arose throughout the years when we needed to find new doctors, since we moved frequently. Sometimes doctors relocated or retired. Occasionally, her symptoms changed, or new symptoms arose, necessitating another new specialist. One time, office personnel referred her to the wrong neurologist, resulting in a horrible experience. Afterward, she refused to see another doctor until prompted by significantly worsening symptoms.

For too many years, new-doctor anxiety resulted from unrealistic expectations. Carole wanted so badly for someone to put a name to what was wrong because she assumed a diagnosis would mean the doctor would know how to fix her problems. She even described *anything and everything* amiss with her body, not differentiating between large and small nor considering oddities everybody encounters from time to time. She theorized that something she mentioned might trigger an "aha" moment for the doctor. Talk about overwhelming them—too much information! It probably also led some to believe mental or emotional issues were involved.

153

It's only within the last few years Carole has changed from looking for a solution to seeking aid to live the best life possible within her limitations. Seeing a new doctor continues to be a stressful experience because of so many strange symptoms, some of which are genuinely weird. In 2014, when her excellent, trusted neurologist retired, a new movement-disorders specialist "coincidentally" moved to Spokane at the same time (we believe God provided this), so there was no break in care. However, this meant seeing yet another new doctor, which meant going back through the records and creating new charts of what happened when.

Charts ease Carole's anxiety when seeing a new doctor. Originally, she used a calendar to record symptoms. Carole first wrote her history on a manual typewriter, then transferred it to a word processor, and finally moved it to Excel. It's easy to add new symptoms, note changes in old ones, and update charts as needed. Now she adapts the chart for each circumstance.

New-Therapist and -Technician Angst
Another area of stress involves seeing a new physical therapist. Since they work from doctors' prescriptions, Carole isn't concerned with preparing a detailed history. This stress stems from the fact her body won't tolerate techniques commonly used to help people overcome injuries or illnesses. If therapists understand and apply that knowledge, they can relieve pain and help her function better. Fortunately, some are open to the challenges posed by neuromuscular impairments, but many aren't. Her worst experience left her unable to walk out of the office unaided. A few don't comprehend the very low level of massage or repetitions her body will tolerate. If they don't learn within a couple visits, she finds someone else. She finds much joy and relief in visiting therapists who do understand and who work within her limitations.

Technicians have also caused problems for Carole. One X-ray

tech refused to listen about positioning challenges and did it her own way, which caused Carole pain for several weeks. In retrospect, Carole realizes she should have insisted the tech pay attention to her needs. Lesson: Stand up for yourself; if necessary, ask for a new technician.

Adventures

Let us each, one and all, give a multitude of hurrahs long and loud for modern medicine! Breakthroughs in knowledge provide many glorious benefits of healing, or at least improvement and help, for storm dwellers as they cope. Some diseases cause people to believe their bodies are out of control. Any relief that alleviates hurts for folks who undergo unending storms of malfunctioning, disabled bodies enables steps into a better quality of life.

At one visit, a physical therapist observed Carole's rowdy back, noting the knotted muscles, and asserted, "Your back is furious today." At times, Carole's battle with her medical trials causes her to feel as if her body is frightfully uncontrolled and angry with her. This physical therapist brought some relief to her.

Our odyssey. Our journey to useful medical care has been long and occasionally frustrating. There have been times when doctors considered Carole prey to imagined physical ailments. The fact she manifested symptoms that didn't completely fit post-polio syndrome confused doctors and complicated matters. One doctor who thoughtfully researched to find a cause for her problems told FJ her symptoms were bizarre. Even today, not all neurological problems are well understood. That doctor who cared enough to search beyond a general awareness of her symptoms exhibited compassion. We remember how he cared for his patients' needs enough to look for the correct answers. Decades came and went before knowledge of Carole's kind of neuromuscular disorders surfaced in the medical field.

The first movement-disorders specialist Carole saw, in 2005, only needed ten minutes in her first appointment to diagnose dystonia, the reason for her strange symptoms. At age fifty-eight, the mystery of lifelong physical limitations such as difficult handwriting, poor posture, and recurrent muscle spasms was solved. What a victory over the fear of an unknown disease; we hadn't known if the outcome would be fatal. Though her strange symptoms can't be cured, she understands why they are present.

In addition to dystonia and post-polio syndrome, Carole has an autoimmune disease which causes various physical afflictions. Someone once asked FJ, "What is wrong with Carole?" To the medically untrained observer, she looks healthy. A few of her unseen effects include leg jerks, involuntary nighttime body arches, weakness, and lack of physical endurance. Sometimes she lapses into semi-consciousness and partial paralysis. Seeing Carole helpless to move is spooky; such episodes are emotionally disconcerting. These hidden physical issues go unnoticed by most people, though members of our family know them well—especially FJ.

Carole now sees a movement-disorders neurologist, a rheumatologist, an ophthalmologist, a pulmonologist, a urologist, and a family practitioner. In addition, she needs physical therapy to relearn correct body mechanics by means of helpful, gentle exercises. Sometimes a physical therapist's back massage helps calm muscle spasms.

Jean and Andy's journey. Medical care fitting the needs of each individual's circumstances is a difficult and puzzling pursuit. Many times, the search for the right doctor takes years. People who have a mixture of afflictions require several doctors, each specializing in one or more areas of study.

We asked Jean and Andy, "What did you experience when searching for medical care? Was the medical care good?" They both burst out laughing. Andy summed it up, "We had pretty good medical care, but we did not have doctors who listened to us." This couple is still seeking answers for Jean's migraine problems that have continued for twenty years—unending storms of stroke-like symptoms, plus diagnoses of fibromyalgia, lupus, psoriatic arthritis, and autoimmune diseases. Every joint is affected, her nerve issues are increasing, and she suffers chronic fatigue. She is now almost completely housebound.

Imagine living in a world of unexpected pain from unknown sources that stresses any part of one's body. Such discomfort disables like an impenetrable curtain hanging between that person and a life of fulfilling important and satisfying goals. Many wind up lamenting to themselves and their families, "I didn't sign up for this."

Gary and Kathy's experience. Kathy had no complaints regarding Gary's medical care. She believes Gary had excellent doctors throughout his long journey.

Jayme and Richard's quest. As a young, smart, and healthy couple, Jayme and Richard traveled together on her downward health spiral. Richard was very passionate and upset concerning Jayme's experiences with doctors. He offers the following observations.

Jayme experienced her symptoms for years before doctors diagnosed the cause. Before the correct diagnosis of Crohn's plus more, medical people told her it was just stress or her imagination. Richard saw strength and pluckiness in Jayme to stand firm in her certainty the problems indicated something was wrong that doctors weren't finding. She stuck up for herself throughout her pre-diagnosis search.

After physicians probed her symptoms and gave their conclusions, she studied the answers given. Richard remembers Jayme's research. "Somebody would tell her something, and she'd spend days or weeks looking stuff up. Sometimes she'd say, 'I don't know where they're getting their information.'" Richard maintains the journey to unraveling the mystery of her illness revealed that knowing and trusting herself was important in telling what she felt inside her body. At last, she found doctors who understood the information she conveyed.

Richard offers advice for the invisibly disabled in their search for answers:

- Keep looking.
- Know and have confidence in yourself.
- Don't accept the answers of "it's just stress" or "it's all in your head."
- Don't accept easy, popular, cover-anything answers; sometimes, doctors just cannot admit they're unable to make a firm diagnosis.
- If the doctors are all about their own agenda, run away.
- Keep looking for a doctor who will look at everything, whether there is just one problem or multiple diagnoses with complications.
- Explore your options to pay for medical care, especially if you don't have insurance. Remember, hospitals have social workers who can help.

In Summary

In the search for medical care to fulfill Carole's needs, we join with others and rejoice long and loud because of the massive amount of research accomplished in recent years. The medical community diligently searches to find cures for the needs of ailing people. In our limited knowledge, it seems wonderful to find medical know-how so readily available. We've spent much time and effort in the search for medical treatment of Carole's symptoms. This pursuit has yielded rewards, including lower pain levels.

Nevertheless, innumerable individuals remain who haven't yet found the help needed for their disabling problems. Why? Because medical research hasn't discovered answers for the myriad of diseases and disorders in existence. When Carole first experienced weird neurological symptoms so many years ago, medical knowledge had only begun to understand her types of disorders. As medicine has reached milestones in movement-disorder research, there remains hope we will see breakthroughs in other areas leading to relief for many others in the invisibly disabled community.

Chapter 12

The Disaster Relief Team—Helpful People

"When you've seen a disaster on the news in the last fifty years, Southern Baptist Disaster Relief (SBDR) volunteers were already on the scene—and they remained long after news cameras left town."
—"Southern Baptist Disaster Relief,"
North American Mission Board

Fourteen years lived in Ione. Skiing. Hunting. Friendships. Ministry. Vacations. Camping. Now it was time to move to Canyonville, Oregon, to begin work in FJ's new pastorate.

Two huge problems hindered the process: one, Carole had neither strength nor endurance to pack everything; two, she lacked the stamina to drive their car on the six-hundred-mile journey. Helpful friends stepped up to support them. Although saddened by FJ and Carole's leaving, women still came to help Carole pack. Hal and Hazel, friends who were planning to travel to visit children in California, volunteered assistance with driving. Hal drove the moving van that towed the Griffitts' car, FJ their pickup and trailer, and Hazel her own car. Carole sometimes rode with FJ and sometimes with Hazel, resting as needed. Although she enjoyed the extra time with her friend, she rued her inability to help.

Disasters and emergencies generate an urgent need for immediate aid. A team of disaster-relief volunteers arrives and provides pressing help. When needs created by the calamity continue for months or even years, disaster relief volunteers become long-term helpers. As teams provide aid during community catastrophes, helpful people assist individuals experiencing disastrous cloudbursts or tornadoes of health difficulties. But when it becomes obvious storms will continue for years, the number of supportive helpers dwindles. They may still be compassionate but can't continue their help. Some doubt the reality of the dweller's situation. Others forget or overlook the person living in Stormyland.

Richard shared his thoughts about people offering ongoing aid. "When you first meet someone, they're willing to help out. But, as they realize you need help and you need it consistently, they recognize it will complicate their lives to help you. They start to avoid you."

Invaluable Comfort

Sufferers need comfort at every stage of adversity. Anyone can offer consolation, encouragement, and reassurance. Renowned preacher Ed Young gives guidance about comforting the hurting in his sermon "Overcoming Tough Times: How NOT to Comfort."[35]

Using the biblical book of Job, Dr. Young analyzes the advice Job's three friends give him. Eliphaz is first to offer comfort. He speaks from his experience: "I know how to do this," or, "According to what I've seen . . ." Bildad expresses tradition: "This is how you handle suffering." Zophar has a bold attitude. He says, "I have this gut feeling," or, "My intuition tells me this." All three played God with Job by telling him—despite evidence to the contrary—he must be a dirty sinner. His wife even told him he should curse God and die.

Dr. Young has seen two types of negative comforters visiting people in the hospital: deniers and wishful thinkers. Deniers seek to comfort by saying, "You aren't going to die," even if it's obviously untrue. The second type may say God told them there will be supernatural healing. Sometimes that is true, but often it's the person's wishful thinking, which isn't helpful to the patient.

Dr. Young does not stop with negatives; he presents positive ways to comfort. One significant recommendation is to show up. Be there with your friend. You need not say much; often, saying nothing is good. Feel as they feel. Don't let yourself be turned off by how they or their house looks or smells. Before Job's three friends began criticizing him, they quietly sat with him doing nothing, just being there. What a comfort!

How can you bring cheer to someone living in Stormyland? Cry with them when appropriate. Cut them some slack, since they're undergoing difficult times. A gentle hug may be appropriate. Don't be judgmental. Be accepting. In most cases, refrain from offering advice. If necessary, speak the truth in love. The book of Proverbs likens a word spoken at the right time to beautiful works of art.

Scripture instructs people in Galatians 6:2, "Carry each other's burdens, and in this way you will fulfill the law of Christ" (NIV). Who in the body of Christ is receiving blessings from God? Those who generously share their lives and abundantly love one another. Part of that sharing includes listening to the needs of others. People who lovingly care for each other exemplify Jesus' love. Those who need comfort and care can seek the prayers of believers in the body of Jesus, the saving Lord of heaven; to do so reveals a humble spirit.

Supportive Churches

People sense God's love through Jesus' body, the church universal. This church is to take God's love to suffering people, including those whose problems are difficult to see. Each member should function as the arms, legs, eyes, ears, and voice of God. If the church neglects this work, how will others learn of God's incredible love for the hurting? The apostle Paul tells us to bear one another's burdens. However, too often, the church avoids those in need; it grows numb and ignores pain signals, "in effect sacrificing a limb of the body of Christ,"[36] damaging itself in the process.

Unfortunately, not all churches nor Christians are sensitive to the needs of the invisibly disabled. Jayme and others we know have experienced being ignored. In a few churches, Carole has also encountered these problems. Individuals in these unhelpful churches didn't consider the needs of hurting people. Many did say, "We'll pray for you." Yet, they never followed through with their actions.

We believe many churches would like to help those living in unending storms; they just don't know how. Perhaps they don't understand the reality and limitations of dwellers. Possibly they don't look past the invisibility to the individual. Maybe their busyness prevents them from helping. Christians need to heed John's admonition in 1 John 3:18 (HCSB): "Little children, we must not love with word or speech, but with truth and action." A church needs to be aware of what is happening in the entire body. Following are some examples of how church people helped us, how church groups aided others, and how individuals and groups can offer help.

164

Practical Help

If light housework is the need, people can collaborate to organize a group. If a volunteer works once a month for two hours, and four volunteers band together doing the same and rotating the weeks, a dweller's house can be cleaned every week. Although each person's time investment would be minimal, the effect for the limited person is monumental. You can apply this pattern to any need the family has: meals, childcare, phone calls, or visits. In this manner, no one person becomes overwhelmed, and yet storm dwellers understand someone cares. In addition, their needs are met.

On a more sacrificial level, a group of sixteen women organized into teams of one pair per shift to help Martha, a twenty-six-year-old woman.[37] She had contracted Lou Gehrig's disease (ALS) less than a year earlier. Her father had died of ALS the previous year and her uncle two years before that, so she knew what to expect. Within three months of her diagnosis, she needed around-the-clock care and had moved into a rehabilitation hospital. With her disease progressing so fast, she had one desire: to have two weeks in her own apartment. The sixteen caregivers and seventeen others who prayed for Martha and her helpers were part of a Christian community who adopted Martha as a project and volunteered everything necessary to fulfill her wish. As a result of their love, Martha lived two weeks in her home and came to God in Christ. Martha wasn't invisibly disabled, and her helpers invested heavily as they rearranged their lives. But this extreme example shows how cooperation can accomplish large projects.

The first time we needed help packing for a move was in 1980 when FJ graduated and we moved to Ione; Carole's boss stepped in, packing our books. Her library experience and expert assistance taught us how to protect our extensive personal library. A double win: help at the time and knowledge for the future.

Some individuals, for various reasons, are highly sensitive to fragrance of any sort. When we visited a large church in another city, we read in the bulletin of their Fragrance-Free Zone—a special room designed for those with chemical sensitivities. It allowed them to enjoy a church service too. A smaller church included this notice in their bulletin: "As a courtesy to others, please refrain from wearing perfume to church." How special that these churches recognized an invisible need. It said to those people, "We see you, we value you, and we support you."

Andy and Jean received help from people in their church. When their boys were small, friends came over to watch them while Jean rested. When needed, some watched the boys while Andy and Jean made emergency room visits. Others helped with practical issues such as household chores and shopping.

In Ione, we were so blessed by the church women who organized annual cleaning events at our house. They shampooed carpets and mopped floors. Cabinets received a thorough cleaning. Women washed walls. Weekly, one woman who lived nearby faithfully cleaned our house. Carole gratefully welcomed her willingness to scrub our bathroom. What a servant's heart! On a lighter note, this friend uncomplainingly pulled down cobwebs Carole pointed out from her viewpoint lying on her daybed. Another woman was always available to call for help on short notice. Altogether, these church women eased our difficult life.

Caregivers Need Help Too

Another area of need inside storms pertains to caregivers. The emotional stresses and physical aspects of caring for a loved one can sometimes overwhelm them. These needs vary according to the limitations of the chronically ill person. Maybe friendship is all the caregivers need. Visits, phone calls, or social media contacts might fill the bill. Perhaps, though, the caregiving is intense, and they require respite time. Someone from the church could fill in for the caregivers while they enjoy shopping or a hobby.

A widow's gratitude. A widow's husband suffered from ALS for eight years, during which her church faithfully supported them. She wrote the following letter to her church.[38] As you read, see what a variety of actions their friends used to encourage and assist this couple.

> Ever since the first symptoms of ALS appeared over eight years ago, you have surrounded us with love and support. You have cheered us with innumerable notes and letters and cards, some hilarious, some profound, some just warm and caring, but all greatly valued.
>
> You visited, and you phoned, often from faraway places. . . . Many of you prepared and brought marvelous food which nourished our spirits as well as our bodies. You shopped and ran errands for us and repaired our broken and out-of-order things while yours waited. You swept and shoveled our walks, brought our mail, dumped our trash. It was possible for us to be a part of our church services because you recorded them. And you brought gifts of love, too many to count, to brighten our hours.
>
> You "doctored" and even repaired a tooth right here in our home. You did ingenious things that made life easier for both of us, like the 'coughing jacket' and signal switch that Norm was able to use until the last few days of his life. You shared Scripture verses with us, and some of you made it your ministry to pray for those who came to our home regularly to give respiratory treatments. You made him feel like he was still a vital part of the music industry and of the church music ministry.
>
> And how you prayed!!! Day after day, month after month, even year after year! Those prayers buoyed us up, lifted us to particularly hard places, gave us

strength that would have been humanly impossible to have, and helped us to reach out on our own for God's resources. Someday we'll understand why Norm's perfect healing did not take place here. But we do know that he was with us much longer and in much better condition than is the norm for an ALS victim. Love is not a strong enough word to tell you how we feel about you!

Norm surely knew he was loved and provided for during his lifetime, and his wife's load was lightened.

Encouraging Friends
Do you know someone who looks healthy yet doesn't fully participate in life activities? Perhaps he or she suffers from an unseen disability. You have the desire to help and support that person; you are compassionate yet busy. So, how can you?

First, seek a friendly relationship, as you would with anyone. A huge problem people with limitations face is a need for acceptance and affirmation. Friendship expresses care and concern and helps ease the isolation many invisibly disabled people experience. Your presence during a visit, phone call, or social media contact affirms their value as a person. Combine those actions with acceptance of their problems, and you provide a sense of self-esteem. However, before visiting, check to be sure they are well enough to enjoy it; find out what time is appropriate. Consider suggesting bringing over lunch, a cup of tea, flowers, or even a video. Remember embarrassment might result because of the messy house they couldn't clean. Do what you can to make them feel comfortable.

A valuable service to offer your friends involves listening to their stories. Their suffering may seem trivial or unreal, but suspend judgment and listen compassionately. Merely recounting what has happened may relieve pressure. Hearing them without judgment affords encouragement. Your friends may be grieving their losses; if so, don't discourage them. Since grief is a natural response to suffering, let yours show. Personal contact is of prime importance in the grieving process. Show your love by being sincerely caring and having a nonjudgmental, non-preachy attitude. Help them focus on the positive and on hope.

If you and your friend are both Christians, perhaps the most important and encouraging support you can offer is to be available to pray whenever your friend has a special need. Sometimes, their plea might just be an urgent "help!" This relationship could develop into mutual prayer support.

How can you help? "Call me if you need anything" isn't the best offer to make, as many people who need ongoing help may not respond. In her book *But You LOOK Good*, Sherrie Connell proposes you call and offer specific help convenient for you. Then your friend doesn't feel guilty for asking you to take time from your busy life. She suggests three possibilities.

- "I am going to the grocery store. Can I pick up a few things for you while I am there?"
- "May I stop by for a short visit with you on Tuesday? Please set aside some towels I can fold or something while I am there!"
- "I need to run some errands. Can I take you to a doctor's appointment while I am out?"[39]

Your ingenuity and depth of compassion are the only limitations on ways to help. Your abilities and available resources may prevent you from carrying out these ideas, but can you network to find others who could? Use these ideas to be a supportive friend.

Finally, remember these two critical needs of your friend: acknowledgment and acceptance as a valuable person, and belief in the reality of the problems.

FJ Reviews

Our disaster relief team throughout the years is long. Faithful friends who interacted with me during the storms of disabling pain as Carole's health slowly spiraled downward. The pray-ers—not the word "prayer" but the people—who, because they cared, prayed both with us and apart from us. And those friends who spent time with us because they—believe it or not—loved us. People who cared about people simply because we are fellow human beings.

I remember a man who befriended me years ago, taking me fishing. We enjoyed a good conversation, and I learned a bit about fishing and the life of my new friend. Today, walks in the pine forests of the Northwest are always therapeutic for me. Time out in nature is like a mini-vacation, bringing a sense of refreshing to my whole being. Sometimes when walking the trail close to home, I meet a fellow sojourner, and we talk about where we are in life. With some who are fellow believers, I engage in a pact to pray for one another.

I vaguely remember part of a song stating the fact people need people. I needed prayer friends, a few fishing friends, some worship-in-church friends, and biological family. Family support is needed during difficult trials; my suffering wife and our children and our parents and siblings have brought joy to my life. Tom and Bill have helped during times of physical hurt for both Carole and me. Carole and our sons share with me a bond of faith in the God of the Bible; this continues to be a strong support for us. "I Enjoy the Trip," sung by the Cathedrals, sums up our feelings. This song captures the happiness and joy of Christian living. When life confuses us with unpleasant surprises, we relate to the song's message that even though things could be better, we enjoy the trip and are happy in the Lord since we walk with Jesus.

Carole Observes

Examples of helpful people abound. For example, Kathy and Gary received help from friends. Some mowed their lawn. Others took Gary fishing. At first, friends and acquaintances encouraged Gary; as time passed, fewer people provided support. Gary wished men would have been more proactive: calling or visiting or inviting him out more often. Gary wanted to reach out, but he was too tired.

FJ and I have experienced help many times from family, friends, acquaintances, and even strangers. I've been grateful when people have opened doors for my wheelchair or scooter in stores, churches, museums, and doctors' offices. Friends have moved chairs at meetings so my wheelchair would fit.

When we encountered vehicle problems on vacations, strangers stopped to help. That meant we didn't have to wait for a tow truck, saving me from total exhaustion. One memorable event occurred on the side of an interstate when our pickup stopped running. We called our insurance company for a tow truck, which arrived quickly. The driver easily fixed our truck, rather than towing it and our trailer back fifty miles to a repair shop, enabling us to get on with our vacation. However, his wasn't the tow truck our insurance company called; he stopped to help us by mistake! Or maybe it was God's Spirit's provision?

Airline flights lasting several hours fatigue me, and I lie across two seats to rest. (I rest my head in FJ's lap.) While on a flight by myself with no place to rest, I explained my predicament to the stewardess. My seatmate offered to move, and our stewardess rewarded him with a move to first class!

People provided transportation for doctors' appointments while FJ still worked.

During and following five of FJ's surgeries and his three strokes, friends brought meals, took me to visit FJ in this hospital, cleaned the house, and provided transportation.

Of greatest importance to me, some people were always available to pray. We often used email and private social media for this.

A special friend offered unique help one Christmastime during my extreme weakness. She addressed and signed all our Christmas cards.

In 2012, FJ and I enjoyed a camping trip back in the Ione area. Our friends Wes and Bonnie picked us up from our campsite and took us to a restaurant to meet other friends, where we enjoyed reminiscing. Unfortunately, I over-exhausted myself. Afterward, too weak to walk unaided, Bonnie helped me to their car. The plans had been to return us to our campsite; instead, they invited FJ and me to their house, so I could rest. My exhaustion soon turned to a severe "spell." Our friends' exceptional hospitality drew the bonds of our friendship even tighter. I rested comfortably and recovered while FJ enjoyed unexpected additional time with friends.

From 1980 to the present, the diverse help and support from family, friends, and even strangers have amazed us.

Chapter 13

Storm Observers—
Friends and Onlookers

"It's bizarre and disorienting when every landmark and
sign your eye knows is suddenly gone, and there's miles
of nothing in its place."
—"The day after, survivors tell
harrowing stories," CNN

*Carole and FJ were exploring Death Valley National Park. Soaking
up the warmth, FJ hiked the trail up to a fantastic view. Too weak
to go with him, Carole stayed in their car with the windows open,
enjoying a breeze and reading her book.*

*Without warning, a terrible laryngospasm hit, almost closing off
her airways, sounding like an asthma attack. Unexpectedly, a stranger
appeared by her window, inquiring if he could help. But she only
shook her head since she couldn't talk. The man stayed with her, gently
talking; his presence comforted her. Soon, she managed to choke out a
request for him to go up the trail and find her husband. Since he was
a professor visiting the park with his students, he sent one after FJ.*

*Carole wondered aloud if he was an angel God had sent. Embar-
rassed, he said anybody would have done it. She glanced around at
all the others and thought, "Well, no one else even noticed." He stayed
with her until FJ hurriedly returned at the fastest run he could manage.*

The man's presence connected her to humanity and made the episode easier to bear.

Can just your presence matter during someone's tough time? You better believe it! Often, the biggest need for dwellers—such as Jayme, Jean, and Gary—is for a friend or family member to understand and support them. They wish for a friend who will be there for them. Sometimes a hug, metaphorical or real, fills the void. Other times, people want a respite from their difficulties; they wish to talk about anything else or to leave the house and go somewhere. Occasionally, a stranger can fill the need.

Storm observers come in various shapes and sizes. They may have any type of relationship, or none, with dwellers. Caregivers, spouses, children, and extended family fill this category. But friends and acquaintances likewise see the storms. Even strangers can witness a need and help, as did the man at Death Valley. These observers do little things, such as moving a chair at church so a wheelchair will fit, and big things like providing ongoing financial help.

Be a Friend

Everyone needs a friend, but the need of invisibly disabled people for compassionate rapport is more pronounced because of their isolation. Relationships with dwellers often appear different than ordinary friendships. Persons with indiscernible disabilities may need adaptive equipment to take part in everyday activities or may be unable to do so at all. They may be unable to participate in social situations because of blindness, weakness, PTSD, or severe depression. However, sympathetic friends can still assist and support.

174

Caring observers naturally want to see their friends' hurts go away. But that will never happen. Their problems won't go away; they can't be fixed or solved, short of a miracle. Observers can seek to gain knowledge about the dweller's illness and provide support without judgment. It helps when they listen, even to tough things. When others give time and space to sufferers who need to rest, it encourages. Offering practical help reinforces friendship.

Carole's idea of a great friend:

> Ideally, she would listen as I vent about a current problem. She would empathize with me over difficulties yet hold me accountable, so I don't over-focus on my challenges. My computer, which I call Expanded World, extends my horizons to life outside my home, but I still need contact with a live person. Therefore, this friend would agree with and respond to what I said in my 1987 testimony: "I do still need your friendship, so please feel free to call or visit—those things don't bother me at all; in fact, they help a lot."

What has friendship looked like for us? In each new town we moved to, at least one woman has befriended and helped Carole. Men were fishing and hunting buddies with FJ. We appreciated help with the house, transportation when needed, and meals brought to us.

Our biggest need from friends is prayer. In our 2014 Christmas card, FJ added this jesting, yet serious, comment. "Dear friends, thank you for your prayers. Please never, ever, no-how, no-way, consider quitting because we are human, so it's a real possibility we always, continually, all the time, every day, every way, need a shield of prayer. If Jesus was tempted in all ways by Satan's traps, it's quite possible we might be too."

Understand Dwellers' Need for Rest

You may see many Stormyland residents sitting or lying down. They may be reading, watching television, or working on their computers. You might fall into the trap of assuming they're choosing to relax—they're just taking a vacation and enjoying themselves. But stop and consider how much you accomplish without even thinking about it. You get up in the morning, get ready for work, continue throughout the day, come home at night, do housework or job-related work or study, eat dinner, and relax before bedtime. Recognize everything involved in completing these tasks. Also, remember you need not stop during the day to rest. Now reflect on just two aspects involved in many types of invisible disabilities: fatigue and weakness. Realize limited persons must choose which few of these many acts they will accomplish in a day. Therefore, don't envy the chronically ill, presuming they're enjoying resting as if it's their choice.

Consider, too, how stressful choosing can be. Who will do essential jobs, such as washing dishes, paying bills, or mowing the lawn? What about very dusty overhead light fixtures? How do activities of daily living get accomplished when weakness or fatigue interferes? Resting is fun, but not when essential tasks are waiting.

Respond Compassionately

Some individuals do act compassionately, such as the professor in Carole's Death Valley experience. Our life has included many sympathetic friends throughout our years of unending storms. We also experienced considerate actions from strangers. Regrettably, though, too often, someone's response is less than helpful. Please note we haven't been recipients of all the following actions and sayings. Unfortunately, many invisibly disabled have. We recognize that when people utter these statements and observations, they may be unaware of potential misunderstandings. Thus, we bring them to your attention and share how we, and others, may react.

It's painful when friends or family accuse the dweller by saying or implying, "It's your fault." If the onlooker regards problems as being caused by the person, he somehow supposes it can't happen to him. He sees no need to be sorry for his friend. Of course, this is faulty logic, but such an attitude still hurts the sufferer.

Chronically ill individuals know many people begin avoiding them when they don't improve. One reason might be they don't want to be around pain. Who does? Not dwellers! An alternative explanation could be an onlooker doesn't accept the reality of the difficulties. Another cause might involve the busyness of onlookers' lives. A different answer concerns how persons perceive the world around them. Often, people see others through the lens of their experience. They conclude, "I was hurting really bad, and I got better. You could too." So, the individual who improved looks down on the one who cannot.

Spiritual motivations also come into play. A Christian may tell a dweller in words or by actions, "I prayed for you, but you didn't get well, so I need not be around you anymore." We endured such an experience soon after Carole's first injury. Carole remembered when two women prayed for her healing, but she wasn't healed, and they refused to come back. Her boss offered an explanation: Christians might fear that if God didn't heal Carole, He might not heal them if they get sick. Consequently, they would be forced into the uncomfortable situation of reevaluating who God is and what He does.

Communicate Thoughtfully

Compassionate people looking into Stormyland from the outside wish to encourage those inside. They want to empathize with dwellers. But often, observers do not understand or realize how their statements and questions may be perceived. Someone living with unending suffering often regards these inquiries differently than those in the everyday, active world. One Facebook group moderator asked what questions, if any, bothered the members. She received swift and extensive feedback. Some reactions to the following sayings may surprise you.

"How are you?" This is a common social conversation opener. But the chronically ill often don't know how to respond. They may automatically say "fine" because they know it's simply a social convention; other times, they react with this word because they know the inquirer doesn't care how they feel. Frequently, they assume the questioner expects them to say they're getting better, even when the person asking should understand the unending nature of their challenges. One woman says she doesn't appreciate that query from someone who does not know her well. A different person answers, "About the same." Still another woman says, "I'm here."

Since strangers, especially, are asking because of politeness, another woman feels they don't need real answers. She also doesn't wish to make them feel awful for asking. She answers with a "fine, thanks" or "nothing noteworthy." She notes friends generally know if she's hurting, so she can be more real.

Caregivers face this quandary too. One such man, Professor Groothuis, whose wife suffers from a serious, progressive condition, gives an unusual answer when asked how he's doing. He says he answers truthfully, "I'm hanging by a thread, but, fortunately, the thread is knit by God."[40] Caregivers may be asked how they're doing, but the inquiry is more frequently about their loved one.

FJ's response: When asked how Carole is doing, I answer, "She's indescribable." If a further inquiry comes, I often reply, "How many hours do you have?" because of the complexity of neurological diseases. Even doctors have a challenge explaining them. Carole's days aren't easily understood by the healthy. Difficult times are common for persons living with several diseases.

178

Such people live with that entity mentioned earlier, the Silent Stalker, who unleashes several sources of pain in their bodies. Days for dwellers in storms of pain aren't usually what could be described as "fine," even when the individual maintains a positive attitude and rarely complains.

Sam Moss, in her blog *My Medical Musings*, offers an in-depth look at this query. She asks, "So how do we, the chronic disease sufferer and the caring friend or family member, live happily ever after with a situation that is ongoing and, let's face it, burdensome to everyone?" She sets it in the context of understanding.

> The chronic disease sufferer needs to understand that people really can't find the right thing to say . . . because what can you say? The caring friend or family member also needs to understand that your response may simply be, "Thanks for asking, still no change," or, "Things are getting a little worse." Depending on who you are talking to, you may feel comfortable to expand with all the gory details.

She sums it up by sharing this important fact: "At the end of the day, contact with others is so important for our overall well-being."[41]

Wayne and Sherri Connell, in their book *But You LOOK Good*, point out it's common for someone whose condition includes pain and weakness to have good and bad days. They suggest asking "how are you feeling?" for those who still have good days and recommend "how are you doing?" when they only have bad days. A seemingly inconsequential difference to an observer, it is meaningful to the dweller. "How are you?" implies either a meaningless social convention or an expected answer of *fine*, or, at least, *getting better.* "How are you feeling?" gives the person a chance to say if it's a good or bad day or to give more information if it's a close relationship. "How are you doing?" says, "I realize you're probably not feeling good, and you may never improve, but are you doing okay in your life today, or are you having extra problems?" Either of these thoughts acknowledges the fact Stormyland dwellers will probably never leave it.

Lori, from a Facebook group, has a different take; she feels "how are you feeling?" or "how are you doing?" are loaded requests. She would rather the questioner make it relevant to the moment by saying, "How is your day?" For her, such a question is easier to answer. Another woman replies about her day, "Oh yeah, pretty easy!" or, "Eh, been worse."

"But you look so good!" Everyone wants to hear they look good. Right? This compliment can backfire with dwellers because, depending on body language or tone, the recipients might interpret it to mean the speaker is implying they must feel good since they look good. Carole says, "I try hard to look good, but how I look has no resemblance to how I feel. Often, when someone says that, I'm feeling especially bad. I seek to remember they mean well, so I thank them and move on." Sam Moss answers, "Thank you. I'm so glad my pain doesn't show through." Or she explains, "It's really important to my well-being that I make an effort with my appearance despite my disease, so thank you for saying that."

A specific observation is better. If you tell your friend she looks pretty or he looks handsome, it will be happily received.

Another version of this question is, "How can you be that sick when you don't even look sick?" Personally, Carole finds this inquiry rude and offensive. It expresses disbelief that the person could be sick. One woman wishes they would rephrase it into a thought such as, "It's such a shame you are so sick, but although I'm sure you feel terrible, let me compliment you. You look beautiful today." What a wonderful comment!

"What are you doing for the rest of the day?" Medical personnel often ask this at the end of a visit. These people should know it may drain the patient just to get to and through the appointment and return home, so they may only plan to rest. When Sam was asked this, she froze for a second. She finally replied, "Nothing. I need to rest after yesterday's appointment and today's podiatry session. It all causes excess pain and disability." After a pause, she followed up with, "My only plans are to write, and I'll be working on my forum." Upon reflection, she wondered why this question affected her negatively. She thinks deep down she still believes she should be living a full and active life. She concluded a better answer would have been, "The rest of my day will be spent resting my body to manage my pain, while writing/blogging and engaging with my Facebook forum members."[42]

"I know what you're going through," or "I know how you feel." Carole sent an email saying this to someone with Parkinson's. This was wrong to say since we don't appreciate it when someone uses these general assumptions with us. People can perceive these phrases as degrading, especially if the onlooker's problem seems slight in comparison. Carole quickly corrected her mistake with a follow-up apology. Here is how the person answered.

> It bothered me many years ago when I would share with someone my wife had cancer, and they would tell me about someone they knew that had cancer, like a brother or sister. I didn't want to be rude, but at that time, when I was struggling to help her survive and to cope with everything, I really couldn't care less about hearing someone else's story about cancer. [She did survive.]
>
> It also bothers me when I hear someone tell someone else with health problems that they know what they are going through, whether it's Parkinson's, cancer, or anything else. It's not possible for me to know what someone else is going through because

I'm not them. Two people that have the exact same symptoms usually have very different experiences because we're all very different, and the way we experience the same things is very different. Anyway, I hate it when I hear someone tell someone else, "I know what you're going through." No, they don't know because they aren't them.

Carole's explanations, when asked how she feels, sometimes lack clarity. She may say her back hurts, or she's tired. She finds it frustrating when the inquirer replies, "Yeah, my back hurts too," or, "I get tired too." Why? She realizes this normal social interaction represents people expressing care and trying to identify with one another. But she finds herself thinking, *Really? Your back actually might hurt worse than mine if it's from disc problems. Alternatively, it might have happened because you sat wrong for an hour. However, does it happen for no discernible reason? Is the spasm so bad you can't sit for even ten minutes? Does the hurt keep you from being active because activity risks further injury? Does it take weeks or months to heal? Has it spasmed repeatedly throughout the years?*

To the response the person is tired, too, her thoughts include these questions: *Does your fatigue last all day long? Are you fatigued by a few minutes of moderate activity, or by ten to twenty minutes of light housekeeping, or by an hour sitting? Do you ever get exhausted when you haven't done anything?* Those are reasons she often passes off inquiries about her health with noncommittal answers.

Dwellers should examine their words and attitudes. Carole realizes it would be better to answer with specifics—for example, "My back spasms are especially painful today." About fatigue, a more effective wording might be, "I'm exhausted even though I've done very little."

When friends respond to her about their physical issues, they might need empathy too. Even when her friends don't dwell in

Stormyland, they can suffer for days, weeks, or longer, and their hurts need to be acknowledged. In addition, she knows she needs to be sure she isn't misjudging the inquirers. In most cases, they do care, or they wouldn't even ask. She also needs to remember her problems are exceedingly difficult to understand.

Andy expresses strong feelings about friends or acquaintances who say to Jean, "I know what you're going through," or, "Yeah, that's my problem too." He says, "One of the things I try—I TRY—to remember is that most people have no clue what's going on. They don't know the depth; they don't know the details; they don't know any of that. I can take their comments poorly, or I can go 'whatever' and move on." He especially dislikes the comment, "Oh, I have migraines too," when they find out Jean has migraines because this condition varies widely in severity. Jean's rare migraines are extremely severe and debilitating, so it sounds as if the speaker is diminishing Jean's struggles. A better practice would be to ask about the other's experiences before trying to identify with them.

Andy and Jean both seek to remember the questioner is trying to be helpful. The person is most likely seeking to show compassion but just doesn't understand how best to express it. They try to remember they can't see what is happening in the inquirer's world.

"Snap out of it" or "quit complaining." This is unhelpful and demeaning. Consider the relative who says, "Just get up and stop being lazy!" Most dwellers' reaction? "As if I could!" Perhaps, "I sure would if I could!" Why would they continue in pain, or stay resting, or remain depressed if they had a choice? Voluntarily enduring painful circumstances indicates serious emotional problems, which is why many consider these sayings insults.

"Just go out and exercise." This comment is related to the previous remarks. Think about the doctor who says to his neurologically weak patient, "Just start walking, and it'll make your back stronger." Carole's reaction: "You don't think I've tried over and

over?" The dweller deems this remark as judgmental because it assumes he's capable but doesn't want to.

Irene, another friend from a Facebook group, has a relative who pushes her to get out of the house. She says, "Oh, but it's so good for you to get out." This relative believes all Irene's fatigability issues are connected to her mental health, and if she just pushes herself enough, she will be well. But if Irene pushes herself, the fatigability will only worsen. These interactions result in Irene avoiding her as much as possible.

"You just need to do . . ." This thought comes in different flavors. One aspect is unsolicited advice: "Have you tried this medication?" or "this specific exercise would help." When Andy says something about Jean's migraines to a friend, he sometimes hears, "Oh, I take this." He thinks, "As if that's all she needs to do!" Does the person not realize she might have already tried that? Or that it may not help her type of migraine?

Another style comes as veiled criticism, meaning "you should try harder!" or "you brought it on yourself!" Those comments will certainly not be received well.

Carole's reflections: Sometimes, a person answers me with platitudes when I share a difficult challenge. My silent rejoinder is *I'm not looking for answers.* After over forty years, I have probably already heard this; I may have even tried it. I just need a hug or to hear, "I care about you." I can courteously share those feelings or just acknowledge that I heard what the person said and go about my day.

Be Careful with Spiritual Observations

Christians should exercise thoughtfulness when talking to or about invisibly disabled people. Above all, God instructs His people to love each other. We can express this love through mutual acceptance and support. Dwellers and observers can help each other. Those enduring ongoing challenges need to exercise care not to be too sensitive to what others say. Onlookers need to consider how dwellers might perceive their words.

"I'll pray for God to heal you." Carole's answers: I say, "Thanks," because we do appreciate and welcome prayers for healing. But if FJ and I are meeting you for the first time, I wonder if you think neither we nor others have ever prayed for my healing. It sometimes leaves the impression you believe your prayers will succeed when no one else's did. Such occasions frustrate us.

A better way for an observer to express his compassion is to ask, "Can I pray for your healing?" I prefer to be asked, "What can I pray for you today?" Such a question gives me a chance to communicate a specific need and let you know where I could use relief and support from God at that time.

"I prayed for you; you should be well." This opinion, unhappily, sometimes follows the offer for healing prayer when the dweller does not get well. Scriptures taken out of context may be included. How would this make a person living with unending illness feel? Sadly, chronically ill people experience this from well-meaning Christians in their churches. This is certainly neither helpful nor loving, and we do not believe it is biblical.

"God won't give you a burden heavier than you can bear." Carole's thoughts: When I hear this, my admittedly selfish reaction is, "God, can't my faith be weaker so You might make the problems lighter?" Or, humorously, "God must sure trust me a lot!"

FJ says: God may not give you more than you can bear, but at times, for purposes we might not understand, the weight seems unbearable. However, I am grateful for divine strength that eventually pulls me through the hard times. Thank you, heavenly Father.

"Just have enough faith, then everything will work out." Carole's ideas: I consider my faith to be deep, but everything is not working out—if, by that, you mean working out "good." How we define good is critical. Acceptance, for me, meant redefining

"good." It does not necessarily mean healing, nor financial gain, nor popularity; to me, it encompasses both end results and what pleases God. "Good" results despite—or even from—hardships. The "good" in my life: My family. This book. My website, Navigating the Storms. Friendships. Deepening of empathy.

A fictional character voices one answer for this: "Having faith doesn't always keep tragedies from happening, but it does make us strong enough to overcome them."[43] Strength and endurance are positive traits resulting from suffering.

The Bible, in Romans 8:28, tells us, "And we know that God causes all things to work together for good to those who love God." This verse shows suffering results in good even when it's hard to see. The life of Joni Eareckson Tada is one example. Joni has been an inspiration to many disabled people and their families because of her tragic diving accident which left her paralyzed from the neck down. Her joy through quadriplegia is contagious. Gary's life, too, is an example. He left a legacy of encouragement for other transplant patients.

"When you're overwhelmed, turn to Jesus." Carole's thoughts: This could fall in the judgmental category; at the least, it's unhelpful. I think, *Okay. This is great advice, but I already turn to Jesus, and He helps me a lot. But the situation is still overwhelming! Now what?*

"God is teaching you something." In Christendom, people commonly speak these words to others in suffering. The unspoken corollary is, once you learn the lesson, your difficulties will end. But what happens to dwellers in Stormyland? An unfortunate truth about being human is we often learn more from hard times than good, but it's wrong to conclude that is the only reason hardship occurs. Therefore, this is a useless observation to make to someone living with invisible disabilities. It becomes hurtful when turned into the question, "What is God trying to teach you?" implying if the chronically ill would just learn their lessons, they would be well.

A related saying, too often heard, is, "God uses the bad times to teach; when you learn, He will restore you." Logical follow-ups by those living in unending storms might include, "Oh yeah?" Perhaps, "Am I so stupid I couldn't learn in all this time?" Another reply from a deep Christian, "That seems rather cruel of God: to take so many years to teach me 'something' when I turn to Him so many times." Or maybe, "I've lived close to God; what have I missed?" People need to keep an open mind when considering reasons unending suffering exists.

"You must have hidden sin." God answers this accusation in the book of Job (42:7) when He responds to Job's comforters that they misrepresented God. Job's friends blame hidden sins for his suffering even though the book's introduction tells the reader Job will suffer because of a spiritual battle. Other reasons exist for suffering than specific, personal sin. Germs. Accidents. Someone else's actions. Situations where no one knows why.

Summing Up

Friends and onlookers, we do not want to discourage you from talking with residents of Stormyland. However, we hope this chapter has given observers insight into ways a Stormyland resident might perceive their conversation. We encourage you to form relationships with the invisibly disabled just as you would with anyone else. Get to know them. Find out their interests. And then enjoy conversations with them.

Chapter 14

Why Storms Exist—Spiritual Questions

"So that you may be sons of your Father who is in heaven;
for He causes His sun to rise on the evil and the good, and
sends rain on the righteous and the unrighteous."
—Matthew 5:45

Suffering severe back spasms, Carole lay quietly on her mom's hide-a-bed. It had been five days since her back-muscle injury, but the pain had not abated. She still could do nothing but exist. That day, her mom brought home two women who volunteered with her in the local Christian homeless shelter. These kindly Christian women wanted to pray for healing for Carole. They prayed, but nothing happened. They left, disgruntled.

As days passed and no healing occurred, they blamed Carole. They told her mom Carole did not have enough faith, or she just would not accept what God wanted for her, or maybe she had some hidden sin. They refused to come again.

What should Carole and her family think? They'd been Christians for years, believing deeply in God and His care. FJ, Tom, and Bill desperately desired to see Carole well again. They prayed for that. So, what was happening? Was it a lack of faith? Did they need to "accept" healing? They'd examined their lives and asked the Holy Spirit to reveal any unconfessed sin. Now what?

A fundamental quandary exists for Christians whose suffering continues for years despite prayers for healing. They wonder, "Why?" Christians hear preachers state, "Just have faith." Others say, "Examine yourself and find your hidden sin." A few television personalities assert, "Simply receive what God has already done for you." Given the abundance of stories about people being healed, these hurting people wonder why they do not receive healing. We've wrestled with this question through four decades. We know God does heal today, but not always. Although we cannot know God's ways and will in all things, we affirm He is good and worthy of our trust.

Telling our story would be incomplete without considering the subject of God, people, and suffering. Many people have authored countless books on this issue, yet no one can fully explain why God allows it.

On the physical level, pain often serves to warn us of danger, an essential and valuable purpose. Feeling a hot stove keeps one from burning his skin more than once. But when people speak about suffering, they usually mean "suffering" from an emotional standpoint. *Why am I suffering? When will God stop my child's hurt? Why does God let my friend's misery continue? How do I navigate unending storms?* Any examination of this question must begin with God, His character, and His plans for people. He created perfection, but He gave His highest creation—humanity—the freedom to choose good or evil.

Origin of Suffering
Suffering caused by painful afflictions did not exist before sin

entered the Garden of Eden, the culmination of God's perfect creation. Why did the sin of rebellion against the Creator enter the dazzling Garden of Eden? When did perfect harmony between the Creator and the created rupture, causing a breach in the loving peace between them? What was rebellion composed of that gave it the power to turn Adam and Eve away from obeying their benevolent Creator?

The first ingredient appeared to be an unusually appealing fellow creature of the Garden, a talking serpent. Perhaps the unique, peerless creature was cloaked with intriguing tropical fish colors and floated effortlessly in the air above the trees, gradually descending until it perched on a tree limb. Eve may have been first to notice the compelling sight, arousing her curiosity and urging her to investigate.

This being, Satan, came to them and presented a spellbinding offer by saying he could show them a different and more appealing way of life than God had given them. He told them they could become like God. He omitted telling them he had already tried to take God's place, and his punishment had resulted in being kicked out of heaven because of his rebellion. The divine Creator had spoken to Adam and Eve saying, "But from the tree of the knowledge of good and evil you shall not eat, for in the day you eat from it you will surely die" (Genesis 2:17). Thus, biblical history records the entrance of suffering that leads to physical and spiritual anguish culminating in death. The entrance of death into the world came through Adam and Eve's willful disobedience to their Creator, the heavenly Father, who created everything that exists in the universe.

Here is one more look at the day of the first couple's mistake relating to the heavenly Lord God. Remember they received a false guarantee when Satan said to Eve something like, "Why not eat from the tree? The fruit looks so inviting." Eve then repeated his words to Adam. This story tells us that although Adam and

Eve did not suffer immediate physical death, pain and suffering entered the world that day. Suffering originated because of the sin of ignoring the word of the Lord of Creation.

Biblical Examples

Job. Be sure not all pain and adversity is caused by the sufferer's sinfulness. The historical account of Job tells us that many thousand years ago, "A man named Job lived in the land of Uz. He was a truly good person, who respected God and refused to do evil" (Job 1:1 CEV). These beginning words describe Job's character. So upright was his moral virtue that Ezekiel 14:14 records God's verbal accolade revealing Job as one of the three most righteous men of all time.

The story continues by telling how Satan brought various afflictions into this righteous man's life. As the narrative progresses, we learn how Job was deprived of family, earthly possessions, and health. We see how his reputation for untainted moral purity was impugned. Even his friends spoke to him, insinuating he was being punished because of evil deeds. His reputation was destroyed because of the suffering and loss of family and possessions. Yet, Job is considered a good man.

Job's trials tested his faith and love for God. Satan, the accuser of all people, asked God whether Job served and loved Him because of the abundant, divinely-given goodies of life: health, wealth, and social favor. Throughout the story, we learn Job's love for God was based on a personal and enduring daily relationship. Job knew life with God was better than life without God. Such is the joy of living.

Job was tested to prove his faith and commitment to God and give testimony that he genuinely loved the Lord because he knew Him. The suffering Job endured while remaining faithful in his love for the Lord is a testimony that knowing God as a friend is more precious than any suffering. Be certain Job cried

192

out for divine healing with an intense longing to receive freedom from his agony.

Hurts bringing emotional, social, physical, and psychological personal malfunctions, whether mild or extreme, began in the Garden of Eden. But determining why someone suffers endlessly is often never clearly known. Perhaps most people have asked why a particular disaster of health, finances, or relationship failure happened to them.

The Apostle Paul. The suffering Paul endured is one most unwelcome by anyone subjected to it. Experiencing a thorn piercing your hand is excruciatingly painful; all you want is the immediate removal of that source of misery. Such an intense pain level is how Paul described what he felt from receiving an unnamed physical torment as a handicap to his work. Paul wrote that he experienced such a physical encumbrance to keep him humble. *The Message*, in 2 Corinthians 12:7–9, records a paraphrase of the apostle's statement.

> Because of the extravagance of those revelations, and so I wouldn't get a big head, I was given the gift of a handicap to keep me in constant touch with my limitations. Satan's angel did his best to get me down; what he in fact did was push me to my knees. No danger then of walking high and mighty! At first I didn't think of it as a gift, and begged God to remove it. Three times I did that, and then He told me,
> "My grace is enough; it's all you need.
> My strength comes into its own in your weakness."

When you are experiencing severe pain, this is a hard answer to hear. There was, however, a greater consolation for Paul: God would sustain Him throughout the handicapping physical affliction. Mrs. Cowman, in *Streams in the Desert*, maintains, "Paul never carried the gloom of a cemetery around with him, but a chorus of victorious praise."[44] Through all his suffering, Paul yet praised God. He knew why he was suffering; he saw how God could get good from it, so he praised.

Lazarus. A man named Lazarus, a very close friend of Jesus, became deathly ill. Lazarus' sisters, Mary and Martha, grew seriously concerned as their brother's sickness worsened. They sent word to Jesus, informing the Lord of his illness. A person might immediately think Jesus would have empathy for such a close friend and quickly command the sickness to leave Lazarus' body. But Jesus was not even slightly fearful for Lazarus' recovery. Because of His perfect understanding of all things, He realized the divine purpose and revealed it to His disciples. "This sickness," Jesus said, "is not to end in death, but for the glory of God, so that the Son of God may be glorified by it" (John 11:4). Four days passed before Jesus arrived at the cave where Lazarus had been buried. At that time, Jesus raised Lazarus from the dead and proved His divinity. Miraculously resurrecting Lazarus displayed His identity as the only begotten Son of God, increasing His disciples' faith.

Habakkuk. Habakkuk's suffering involved watching his country be invaded by an evil enemy, the Chaldeans. He knew God allowed this as punishment for Israel's sins. Yet, he pleaded with God to relent. This little-known prophet prayed for relief and received God's answer. It was *no; Israel has sinned too much, and God will not change His mind.*

This book is the ultimate example concerning God's sovereignty because Habakkuk never saw the good that would come from the bad. Job's trials ended, and he received great blessings. God was with Paul and strengthened him, enabling him to do great things for God. Lazarus was brought back to life. But in Habakkuk's time, Israel received the punishment of being overrun by her enemy. And yet Habakkuk ended with this prayer of absolute trust in God in Habakkuk 3:17–18.

> Though the fig tree should not blossom
> And there be no fruit on the vines,
> Though the yield of the olive should fail
> And the fields produce no food,
> Though the flock should be cut off from the fold
> And there be no cattle in the stalls,
> Yet I will exult in the LORD,
> I will rejoice in the God of my salvation.

God's Sovereignty

What does *sovereignty* mean? And how does it pertain to God? Sovereignty means *to have supreme authority or power*. Synonyms include dominance, jurisdiction, and supremacy. As applied to God, these mean God has absolute authority and dominion over everything imaginable. He has perfect freedom and, therefore, the power to do whatever He chooses. No one or no thing is more powerful than God. We created beings cannot dictate to Him. Remember, though, God has immeasurable love for His creation.

Which begs the question: With all this power and love, why does God allow suffering to continue? There is a false premise prevalent in today's thinking. Many people assume only two views exist about God and suffering. One belief says God is powerful but does not care if a person hurts. The other opinion says God cares and is sorry that humans hurt, but He is impotent and cannot do anything about it. However, we believe the answer has to be this: It's beyond our understanding. God IS good. And God IS powerful. God also loves us beyond our comprehension. But for reasons known only to Himself, God has let hurtful things happen; He lets these things continue to happen. Despite humanity's unworthiness, God still displays His sovereignty by His love for people.

Suffering Today

Since God created everything perfect, no evil existed, no harmful germs lived, and no genetic defects happened. These all resulted from man's rejection of God. So now, as throughout history, the good person suffers along with the evil person. In addition, sometimes bad things just happen. Our bodies grow weak; they are subject to germs; they have genetic defects; they age. In these cases, nobody did anything wrong; we are not being punished. No satisfactory answers exist.

Lysa Terkeurst says, "I make such big assumptions of what a good God should do and then find myself especially disappointed when the winds change, the struggle bus takes a sharp turn left, and nothing at all feels right."[45] We have all expected God to do good, yet distressing things have happened. This is the heart of the issue concerning God, sovereignty, and suffering. We wonder if God has a right to do whatever He decides to with our lives. If He can do or even allow unpleasantness—things that look wrong to us—to happen in our lives, does that make Him a bad God? If He does allow suffering, can we continue to love Him? Is He still worthy of that love?

The apostle Paul answered this with a resounding yes! He praised God during all his suffering because he knew God is both good and great. His life exemplified a confidence that it did not matter what he suffered when other people saw God and accepted Jesus as a result.

Even amidst suffering, God gives enough strength to enable people to fulfill His plans for them. Disabilities cannot prevent individuals from accomplishing what God desires for them to do.

Suffering can produce unexpected strengths: resilience, endurance, and maturity. When men and women weather hard times, these unanticipated traits develop. These attributes should be practiced with a victorious spirit, not whining or complaining. When Christians suffer yet do not deny God, they are in effect saying, "God is worth everything. He is more important than my suffering. God is so, well, *God* that compared to knowing Him, my pain no longer matters."

Unfortunately, some people ascribe poor explanations for problem times. Some say all suffering is to make us usable. Such a belief implies that without suffering, we could accomplish nothing for God. Another unfortunate idea says this is all to teach us something, indicating there is no other way to learn. A similar claim is we learn from suffering. While that may be true, we can learn good lessons in other ways. Still, another argument says our suffering shows God's love when, like a railroad track switch, the difficulties change the direction of a person's life to a more productive path. Joni Eareckson Tada says the good that God has accomplished through her life outweighs her suffering. However, we can see the example of Christians such as J. C. Penney, founder of the department store of the same name, and R. G. LeTourneau, prolific inventor of earthmoving equipment and Christian philanthropist; their lives demonstrate that suffering is not always necessary for success.

Contemporary Examples

People who maintain loving faith and service to God during their time of hurt give witness to the reality of divine love being poured into their spirit. Contemporary examples exist of hopeful, productive living despite unending disabilities. Some stories seem miraculous, but these successes may require a strong resolve and tremendous exertion to attain.

Joni Eareckson Tada is one who exemplifies a life of hope and inspiration for millions of disabled people. Paralyzed at seventeen, she eventually learned how to make use of her quadriplegia in astonishing ways. Through tremendous effort, she became an artist, producing beautiful art by holding a paintbrush in her mouth. She has authored multiple books. She founded Joni and Friends (JAF) with various national and international ministries for and about disabled people. JAF promotes Wheels for the World, globally providing mobility for people. The organization also sponsors national and international camps for the disabled and their families. It produces radio and television series, and it established The Christian Institute on Disability. This organization was founded by a disabled person living a life of hope and purpose. Even though Joni is not invisibly disabled, she remains an example of why God sometimes does not heal and how He can work through a willing person.

George Matheson, born in 1842, became a well-known preacher in Scotland. With poor, blurry vision from birth, he nevertheless pursued education, earning his master's degree. He was pastor of several churches. His virtual blindness was unknown by his parishioners and the people around him. This invisible disability led him to his knees. Praying the following, as Matheson did in his work called *Moments on the Mount*, is never easy.

> My God, I have never thanked Thee for my thorn. I have thanked Thee a thousand times for my roses, but not once for my thorn. I have been looking forward to a world where I shall get compensation for my cross as itself a present glory. Thou Divine Love, whose human path has been perfected through sufferings, teach me the glory of my cross, teach me the value of my thorn. Show me that I have climbed to Thee by the path of pain. Show me that my tears have made my rainbow.

Countless people live today, nameless except to God, who wrestle with their invisible disabilities. They pray and cry out to

God for relief, but in the end, they praise God for who He is and for His presence and strengthening.

Thoughts about Healing

Another question people who do not get healed wrestle with is, "If You are all-powerful and You don't heal me, then doesn't that imply You *want* me to hurt?" Does God WANT a person to hurt? The answer depends on what "want" means. When a child needs surgery, the parents want him to have it because they realize the outcome will be worth the ordeal. God knows more than we can possibly understand, so even when we suffer unendingly, God must know the outcome will be worthwhile.

When thinking about her difficulties, Carole says, at times, "I want it over, like NOW." We know it can be hard to discern what is from God, especially when it's difficult to accept. Carole admits that buried deep inside is a hurt, maybe anger, that God heals others, but He does not heal her. People who believe God heals ALL sickness often say, "God can do all things," meaning God will always heal. But Carole responds, "Yes. He CAN do all things, including strengthening me through these challenges. Which is harder for God: healing or strengthening?"

Yes, these bodies are ours, but they are also the temple of the Holy Spirit. Therefore, not being healed becomes God's responsibility. And we trust Him because He is good. Do we believe God or turn away and try to live life on our own, which leaves us with no comfort, no hope of future healing, and no heaven to anticipate?

Some may wonder if God even cares about them in their struggles. The proof that He does is shown by Jesus' life, death, and resurrection. God loved people so much He sent His only Son into the world to provide a way for people to spend eternity with Him if they choose. Garrett, in the novel called *Vanishing Point*, puts it well: "And what I'm realizing is that when he doesn't intervene, it doesn't mean that he isn't there. I think it means just the opposite. He decided not to just sweep down and fix our problems every time something goes wrong. Instead, He chose to redeem us eternally by sending His Son."[46]

In light of God's love, why wouldn't healing me be a good thing? The answer lies in a person's perspective: Who is God? And how important is He? One author, Ralph Muncaster, believes, "We must ultimately realize that God is in control—and that God is loving, God is just, and God is holy. His acts of love, justice, and holiness have been documented over thousands of years. We aren't in a position to judge Him. The final answers to suffering lie in a dimension beyond ours—because they lie with God Himself."[47]

When healing doesn't happen, people often try to understand what cannot be understood. They can doubt what God says in the Bible. In a novel called *The Healer*, an older Christian speaks to a newer Christian whose sister is dying from cancer. The young Christian is perplexed, upset, and doubting. "'Christianity isn't what you thought it would be like. Okay. So change your expectations.'"[48]

When reading about the awfulness of Jerry Sittser's grief about his family members' deaths, for the first time Carole realized we Christians pick and choose the painful areas of life we expect God to remove. Some people teach that a person just needs faith to be healed, find a job, or receive money, but then ignore areas such as a loved one's death or other permanent losses—an ex-spouse who has remarried, a repossessed house that has been sold. We don't expect dead people to come alive, so why do we assume God will always heal if we just "have enough faith"?

Conclusion

The fundamental belief underlying our choices remains this: God is good, He is powerful, and He loves us beyond measure. How do we explain unending suffering in this world? We cannot. We are unable to account fully for why God sometimes heals but often does not.

Theologians throughout the ages have sought to find a comprehensive answer for this question but have failed. An answer exists, but it mystifies people. Isaiah 55:8–9 describes what God says:

> "For My thoughts are not your thoughts,
> Nor are your ways My ways," declares the LORD.
> "For as the heavens are higher than the earth,
> So are My ways higher than your ways
> And My thoughts than your thoughts."

These verses may make God appear strange or even terrible. However, if God is a good Creator, He has the ability and power to think and act differently than the created.

Romans 8:28 adds another dimension. "And we know that God causes all things to work together for good to those who love God, to those who are called according to His purpose." And Jeremiah 29:11 tells us, "'For I know the plans I have for you,' declares the LORD, 'plans to prosper you and not to harm you, plans to give you hope and a future'" (NIV). When we consider these verses from Isaiah, Romans, and Jeremiah, along with God's character, trusting God in difficult circumstances seems a reasonable approach to adopt in life. Therefore, we choose to trust Him—His goodness, His power, His love—and love Him in return.

Chapter 15

When Storms Get Personal—
Spiritual Applications

"The sufferings of life are God's winds. Sometimes
they blow against us and are very strong. They are His
hurricanes, taking our lives to higher levels,
toward His heavens."
—L. B. Cowman, *Streams in the Desert*

When darkness seems to hide His face,
I rest on His unchanging grace;
In ev'ry high and stormy gale,
My anchor holds within the veil.

On Christ, the solid Rock, I stand;
All other ground is sinking sand,
All other ground is sinking sand.[49]

How do you live when your problem is not removed? What
emotions do you wrestle with when it appears God ignores
you? What is your response to added new symptoms or diagnoses?

How can you live with your life as it is while still believing God heals today? If God heals today, why doesn't He heal you? If He truly loves you, He would heal you, right?

These questions recur with each new or worsening storm, requiring attention yet again. We struggle with these dilemmas. But, again and again, we return to this conclusion: Jesus is sufficient. The words of the old hymn "The Solid Rock" sum up our experiences admirably.

More questions emerge. Where does a person go when faced with an unpleasant health diagnosis? Where is the road leading from that tossing, turbulent life we were thrown into? What became of the peaceful existence that morphed into a disastrous emotional maelstrom? Sometimes disabled people perceive their wall of inability to be an impenetrable barrier they can't get through to find life feasible and reasonable to grasp. What is the way enabling them to emerge into peace and victory over their plight? How does anyone cope with such heartache, pain, or stress the invisibly disabled endure? There must be an answer enabling them to thrive successfully in their new restricted lifestyle. Many who endure recurrent, unending storms puzzle over these thoughts. FJ has heard their pleas for deliverance from their situations. These people need the ability to cope during ongoing storms. We find this strength through our relationship with God.

So we spend time, as do others, in the following areas as we cope with our circumstances when an all-knowing, all-loving, all-powerful God does not heal us.

Loving God When There Is No Change
Looking to who God is. These questions have no answer apart from who God is. He has more knowledge than we have. He sees more than we can. He knows our end from our beginning, including our journey and pitfalls along the way. Thus, He thinks

and acts differently than we do. But He loves and cares for us more than we can imagine.

Sometimes, the darkness appears impenetrable, seemingly so dark even God can't enter. In those times, we need to "judge the present by the future."[50] We remember who He is and what He has done. And we look forward to the future He has planned for people: heaven.

Your view of who He is will determine how you perceive hurtful things. If you are the sufferer, talk to God about your anguish. Be honest. Ask for comfort. Do not bargain. Do not demand. Approach Him as a loved child. Focus your thoughts on things that are true, noble, right, pure, lovely, and admirable (Philippians 4:8). Recognize God has allowed these difficulties for His purpose. The essential question is this: Do we trust God or not?

Appreciating the joy of music. FJ remembers working in a geriatric ward and observing a lady who lay in her room, dying. She surprised him by singing hymns of faith: faith in the Lord of heaven and in her final destiny. She sang with clarity and confidence. Three days later, she had gone from the troubles and trials of this earthly life to a joyous eternal existence. This elderly lady had hope based on faith in the God described in the Holy Bible. Facing death didn't change her belief in God's promise that Jesus had paid the death penalty for all who fall short of the way God originally intended people to live. This was one elderly person's means for coping with her circumstances. There was neither fear nor worry for this lady because she believed what the Bible says: by grace through faith in Jesus, she would gain eternal life. She sang with the joy found only through faith that Jesus saves for all eternity.

Music has captured every situation—of joy and sorrow and of triumph and tragedy. FJ finds gospel hymns and songs best for coping with life. We include Christian songs as part of our devotion time, for they tell of divine help that lifts our spirits, and they encourage us with spiritual truths. The act of singing releases us from the sorrow of discouragement and opens the spirit to joy. Music reminds us of precious lessons that have encouraged us in pleasant and difficult times. Joyful music defeats hopelessness that brings lethargy and renews faith in the possibility of improvement. Music of faith affects mental attitude, creating a more positive outlook on life. A special favorite is "His Eye Is on The Sparrow." Positive words and a happy melody lift the spirit, bringing a satisfying mood.

Carole finds music a comforting source to soothe her, especially during times of intense pain. There have been sleepless hours during unending episodes when her body just feels indescribably wrong. She listens to music portraying the beauty of Christianity—quiet songs sung about overcoming. Music has the power to soothe and enable her to experience inner calm despite pain. When FJ was in rehab following his second mild stroke, she repeatedly played "We'll Not Be Defeated," sung by Dale and Rita Lidstrom. It reminded her of God's sustaining power and enabled her to believe in FJ's return to health.

Sometimes when you hear a song, God adapts it to your need, whatever it may be on that day. While listening to John Denver's song "Some Days Are Diamonds," FJ received thoughts from God that he used to compose a poem. He speaks of wonderful days, like diamonds, and tough days, like stones. He brings in God's presence, repentance, and cleansing. But FJ finds his answers to the hard times in Psalms. Part of his poem follows:

> But I add the psalmist's words and mine,
> "The Lord is my Shepherd." I follow Him; that's
>   where I belong
> Those days of hurt and pain, guilt, and shame
> These are heart stones that make my spirit groan.

When days weigh down your soul like rough, dull,
    hard stones
Remember Immanuel—God with us
He died that I might turn from sin to right and be
    where I belong
At last, my stubborn will bends in anguish on
    bended knee
Immanuel said, "Come take abundant life
    with Me."
He's been saying every day of history,
"Come to me where you belong."

FJ Griffitts

All these thoughts resulted from listening to music. And even though he applies these reflections specifically to being in tune with God, they can also apply to living in storms. "Heart stones" aptly describes our challenges. We remember God gives us abundant life too. We know some days are God's diamonds, but some days feel like a stone.

FJ enjoys an eclectic music taste. He appreciates John Denver's songs along with a variety of other singers. But we both find encouragement through hearing Christian vocalists who bring joy and comfort through their music. Bill and Gloria Gaither are among many Christian singers who entertain and bring spiritual food for the soul. Singing along with them encourages the deep-down-inside person.

Singing favorite songs. Music provides an excellent way to cope. Passively listening to it relaxes us. Singing or humming songs we know and love actively helps us thrive during rainy times. "There's Something About That Name" by the Gaithers speaks about the sweet smell following a rain, reminding us good can follow unpleasant. The Negro spiritual "He's Got the Whole

World" tells us, "He's got the wind and the rain in His hands," pointing out God is in control even when we dislike what we see.

"Sunshine in My Soul" prompts us to remember we can be happy despite our circumstances. A contemporary song, "Blessed Be Your Name," has a verse reminding us we can bless God's name even during times of pain and suffering. Carole finds this idea particularly poignant. Sometimes, it seems her challenges are too much to bear. She knows she has no choice in the matter, but she acknowledges God does. Again, she wonders why He doesn't heal her. But she ends up surrendering her life anew to God, honoring Him and recognizing He is worthy of all praise regardless of what happens to her. The song also speaks of God taking away and giving. Carole's first thoughts revolve around all that has been taken away in her life, but then she remembers everything given to her: FJ, Tom, Bill, their families, and her close friends.

So, singing favorite songs, even off-key, provides an excellent coping mechanism.

Applying the truth of Scripture. Reading, studying, memorizing, and meditating on Scripture is an integral part of our lives. Since we deem it to be the Word of God, how can we ignore it? Below are Scriptures that encourage us, hold us up in hard times, give us direction, or tell us more about God.

- Second Corinthians 12:9 reassures us God can use anything in our lives. "And He has said to me, 'My grace is sufficient for you, for power is perfected in weakness.' Most gladly, therefore, I will rather boast about my weaknesses, so that the power of Christ may dwell in me."
- First John 5:14–15 can be applied to the question of healing. It talks of having confidence in God and asking for anything according to His will.

Hence, we know whatever His will is, He will carry it out. So, Carole prays, "Be it done unto my body according to Your perfect will." She rests in assurance that He loves her and will carry her through whatever He deems best.

- Isaiah 55:8–9 tells us God's thoughts and ways are different and higher than ours. So, we can rest in the thought His plans are excellent.
- Isaiah 43:2 surprises us as it says, "When you pass through the waters, I will be with you; and through the rivers, they will not overflow you. When you walk through the fire, you will not be scorched, nor will the flame burn you." God Himself says in this verse He is delivering through, not from, these hard situations. In addition, He says He will be with us. What a comfort!
- Philippians 4:6–7 speaks of the wonderful peace of God that surpasses all our understanding. But we note this peace comes with submission of everything to Him in prayer. This implies absolute trust in God. We give the problem to Him, knowing He will take care of it.

FJ notes Carole finds comfort and inner strength as she reads and ponders Scripture. She savors an early morning devotion. Shortly after waking, she's busy reading the Bible and spending time prayerfully listening to the Holy Spirit. These times are part of her personal relationship with the heavenly Father. They strengthen and enable her to have hope despite her life of pain. Her faith that God loves her grows stronger because she feels Him holding her in His hand. Her inner strength enables her to cope with the adversity of multiple challenges.

We recommend teaching young children the importance of

knowing the Bible. We base this on FJ's childhood experiences. He relates that reading the Bible has been a help since he first learned to read. When he was a young boy, his church held a weekly Bible study at different members' homes each week. Everyone sat in a circle as each person, including children, read a verse of Scripture. Adults encouraged children to do their best, helping them with unfamiliar words. In these studies, FJ learned to read at an early age and gained familiarity with the Bible. FJ draws encouragement and comfort from awareness of this book he believes is the Word of God. Abraham Lincoln said to a friend, Joshua Speed, concerning the Bible, "Take all this book upon reason that you can, and the balance on faith, and you will live and die a better man."[51]

Carole read an article that stands strong in her memory. Though the specific article is lost in the history of things once read, its threefold thesis talked of "if, because, and even though." The author concluded: *If* God does this, then I will love Him. *Because* God did this, I love Him. *Even though* God lets awful things happen, I will still love Him. These thoughts stayed with her because of her increasing limitations. Habakkuk 3:17–18 states a worst-case scenario. The prophet had been told God would let invaders bring horrendous disasters, yet Habakkuk responds he will still exalt and rejoice in the Lord.

Invoking the power of prayer. For many people in troublesome times, prayer is a coping mechanism. It brings relief from feeling over-stressed and emotionally drained. When individuals wear out from incessant pain, or they become run-down mentally or emotionally, unable to continue grappling with multiple assaults, prayer often brings peaceful relief. When days of unending trial come along, those who have been praying and keeping up their inner spiritual strength have an added ability to endure. On rainbow days, when people feel ecstatic, thinking life cannot get any better, prayer is also in order—thankful prayer. Since some periods of life are jubilant, stable, and pleasant, they should include praise to the heavenly Father. God responds to people who know Him and are thankful enough to express their gratitude in praise for His goodness.

Faithful church attenders likely know how to act when a prayer's answer is yes, no, or wait. But how do we react when God is silent? Or when no answer comes? Do we resort to begging God? If so, what are we really saying? Aren't we saying we should be exempt from the human condition? Because we belong to God, do we expect Him to take away the terrible things that happen to all people? We need to remember Matthew 5:45: "For He causes His sun to rise on the evil and the good, and sends rain on the righteous and the unrighteous." We aren't exempt from bad things just because we may be righteous people.

Instead of begging God, we may try to manipulate Him through our prayers. Too much teaching on prayer demands specific answers from God or even borders on manipulation: *If we do such-and-such, God will do this.* As humans, we want what we want when we want it. God hasn't healed Carole, and she doesn't understand why. But she says God is God, and she is not. She must have faith God is a loving and powerful God who has excellent reasons to allow what He does.

Another issue of prayer that bothers Carole is asking others to pray. When she undergoes turbulent, stormy days, she instinctively wants friends to lift her up. However, sometimes she wonders if she does it for the right reasons. Maybe she assumes the number of people will persuade God to quiet the tempests. Or possibly she imagines God will pay greater attention to a more spiritually mature person. Nevertheless, she reaches out to ask others to pray for specific needs and frequently receives calmer weather.

Praying for another's healing is a thorny issue. When we don't receive healing, do we find it difficult to pray for someone else to be healed? Carole does. She has no problem asking God to heal that person, but she has immense difficulty believing the Lord will, even when she longs for the person to be well. She wrote this prayer: "Because of my increasing challenges, which I believe You allow for Your reasons, I find it difficult to pray for others' healing, expecting You will do it. Since my experience is that Your will isn't always what people call 'good,' I wonder if Your will for whom I pray might not be 'good' either. Help me, Lord, to have discernment to pray Your will. Help me, also, to not expect (or be afraid) You will let the 'bad' happen."

Joining with others in worship. We find joy in the presence of the heavenly Father; He has been so good in providing freedom to join with other Christians in worship. Attending where we have friends in Jesus brings joy and encouragement into both our lives. The blessing of friends we share life with causes us to offer thanks and praise to God for them.

Expressing heartfelt praise. But how can we praise during these hard times? We should take a cue from birds and plants that thrive amidst inhospitable environments. Birds fly through the storm's winds, rising against the turbulence. Several flower species grow and flourish in alpine conditions. As in the natural realm, tough times can provide a stimulus for growth. That alone is a reason for praise.

We base the need for praise on 1 Thessalonians 5:16–18, which tells us to rejoice and give thanks. We can praise in both good and bad times. Even on rough days, we can usually find positive things to give thanks for. We can also praise God for His presence during our challenges. Carole wonders if she should call gray days "ugly" since the Lord also creates them, and they may serve a positive purpose. She asks God to help her find the proper perspective between being happy *for* storms (unrealistic) and seeing them *only* as ugly or bad (unhelpful). There are two extremes of viewing our storms: being happy for bad things or bitter about them. Either makes coping harder.

It's good to thank God for being the Weather-Maker, both in the world and in our lives. We should be thankful—not for the pain—but because He, the almighty, all-powerful, all-loving Creator, made that decision for His reasons. He set rules in place that govern the world's weather, though sometimes He overrides those laws of nature and changes them. He also does this regarding physical storms: He sets in motion how our bodies operate, yet sometimes He steps in and voids those rules.

We also offer praise for creation. Worshiping the heavenly Father and having an awareness of heaven and earth—even the entire universe—is a delight. An endless mystery exists concerning the intricacy of the human body. What a wonder of creation the brain is! "A typical healthy human brain contains about 200 billion nerve cells, or neurons, linked to one another via hundreds of trillions of tiny contacts called synapses."[52] We have difficulty envisioning a billion of anything. But two hundred billion nerve cells, just in the brain? In his book *Beyond a Reasonable Doubt*, Dr. Frank Harber suggests it requires more faith to believe this miracle just "happened" than to accept God exists and designed the human body.

In FJ's high school days of being a less-than-avid biology student, he found he actually enjoyed reading descriptions of desert plants when they were written by author Zane Grey in his books about the American West. FJ's teacher, Mr. Finney, was not impressed with FJ's choice of "textbook"; FJ realized the extent of his teacher's displeasure when his report card arrived with a lower-than-low grade. He still finds westerns more thrilling than biology but enjoys Dr. Frank Harber's book called *Beyond Reasonable Doubt*, where he describes fascinating information about the human eye. Harber writes, "The eye contains 130,000,000 light-sensitive rods and cones which generate photochemical reactions that convert light into electrical impulses. An incredible one billion such impulses are transmitted to the brain every second."[53] Dr. Harber presents extensive, convincing scientific evidence pointing to a beneficent Creator—God. We give thanks and praise because the heavenly Father of life endowed the human body with a matchless biology and spirit.

Experiencing the solace of nature. A poet describes times of utter despair and how he overcomes despondency by going into nature. "I come into the peace of wild things who do not tax their lives with forethought of grief."[54] He returns to his world feeling peaceful. A walk along our local trail brings FJ peace. We deeply love nature because God created it and called it good. Walking on a trail through varieties of trees, flowers, and shrubs is like a short relaxing vacation to FJ. He derives great pleasure in hiking a trail, viewing a landscape of flowers, or exploring a cactus garden—a favorite delight of his.

For people who can't walk, there are wheelchairs and electric scooters to use on accessible trails. There are other ways to view nature for homebound individuals, such as DVDs that showcase creation's artistry in our national and state parks and contain many splendid sights. Whenever we visit a park gift shop, we pick up a DVD to enjoy later. These DVDs are also available online.

We worship the One with the power to create nature's wonders; we appreciate the resulting marvels.

Pursuing comfort from God. God brings comfort in times of distress. Jesus' presence provides the ability and strength to thrive amidst storms. But God also brings comfort through others—family, friends, acquaintances, coworkers, schoolmates, and even strangers. God knows no limit as He comforts us.

Carole asserts, concerning her difficulties, that her goal is to make lemonade from the lemons in her life. How can she do that? She strongly believes spiritual comfort flows into her from feeling God's presence. Neither of us has an answer for why some people live lives of suffering. Carole possesses an assurance that God cares for and walks with those who can say with Romans

8:38–39: "I am sure that nothing can separate us from God's love—not life or death, not angels or spirits, not the present or the future, and not powers above or powers below. Nothing in all creation can separate us from God's love for us in Christ Jesus our Lord!" (CEV). Because God reaches out in love to her, Carole drinks sweet lemonade as she reaches up to God in heaven.

Carole's testimony. The following talk was presented to Ione Baptist Church at the morning worship service on January 18, 1987. FJ subsequently printed it in the monthly newsletter.

> Most of you know me, but what you may not realize is how very weak I am and growing weaker still. Much of my life is spent in restoring my energy (resting, not sleeping) so I can function somewhat normally. You usually see me at church because I want very much to be able to worship and learn with God's people, and God honors that with the extra strength needed to stay up for so long a time. I praise Him for this. I do still need your friendship, so please feel free to call or visit—those things don't bother me at all; in fact, they help a lot.
>
> I've only said these things to give you a perspective on the testimony I feel called to share with you this morning.
>
> GOD IS NOT JUST A MEANS TO AN END; GOD *IS* THE END. What I mean is Christian living and doing God's will is NOT just a means to a contented, fulfilled life. Living for God IS important, but God Himself is the whole reason for existence. He created the world; He redeemed people, and He sustains everything. His love—who He is—is what gives life meaning. His love is enough. Whatever I have to go through is endurable because *He loves me.*

This past week, these thoughts have taken on new significance for me. For if these thoughts are true, and they are, the only response I can give is that my life should be wholly given to Him in gratitude.

He means so much to me, first, that I willingly give an "OK" to whatever He allows to happen in my life, even if it is (and continues to be) painful. That was a hard lesson for me to learn because I don't want to hurt. I want to be strong again. But He loves me so much He would not allow this if there were any other way. (Please understand I refer to circumstances beyond my control, not those which are a result of my sin.)

Second, giving my life to God in gratitude means I seek what He wants me to be with my life and not just *do* whatever I have the ability to do. I used to *do* whatever needed doing that I could do, and many times that is the way God leads people, but He wants so much more. He wants my very will to want Him and His purposes for my life, not just my activities.

Third, it means when I can't *do* anything at all and don't know what He wants me to do, I'll fill my life with seeking Him and just soaking up His love. For me, that includes reading, studying, and memorizing His Word, praising, praying, interceding or meditating, or just listening to songs about Him. And that's been a beautiful time this week.

One of my regrets, though, is I didn't come to this place of surrender while I still had my strength to offer this Lord who loves me. I only came to know and do these things after I only had weakness left to offer my God—the One who makes my life worth living.

I thank God now for this church, the people in it, and the experiences I've had in Ione that have helped me to come to this place. And for the further experiences awaiting me.

My prayer for you is, don't wait to learn God is *not* just the means to an end—He's *not* just the way to a contented, fulfilled life. He *IS* the end—your whole reason for being in life.

"Praise the Lord!"

Clinging to Trust in God

Trusting God because He understands suffering. People demand that God come experience pain and suffering, but in Jesus, He already did! Since Jesus, as a human, endured suffering, we know God understands hurt. By His response, we recognize God suffers with us through the cross; in that experience, Jesus also felt forsaken by God.

When Jesus came to our world, He experienced life in human form. By His suffering, He demonstrated God's incredible love for us. People didn't expect Jesus, the Son of God, to die, so His death reveals that people don't always comprehend God's plans. His suffering and death provide for our future life. His incarnation, life, death, and resurrection offer Christians reasons to live and thrive, even during times of suffering. It gives Christians resources to cope with their suffering that others don't possess.

Defining trust in actions. Kathy emailed this to us before Gary passed on to glory:

God is letting us go through some experiences that we have no control over. I don't like the situation, so I have to trust God's plan. Maybe I'll get to see the outcome; maybe I won't. Only He knows what's going on. But I still choose to serve Him and to

217

wait for His plan to unfold, and I know you are too.
Ohhh, I still have my fits now and then and get all
huffy, and He knows that. But after throwing my fit
and then asking forgiveness, I feel better.

Trust, for us, means believing God has His reasons for not
healing Carole. If God doesn't exist, her suffering is a fluke, and
she has no heaven to look forward to. If He is a powerless God,
then why should we trust Him at all? If He can't help, again, we
have no hope. If He just doesn't care, what can we cling to?

A fictional character whose mother died in an accident spoke
these words about trusting God: "'It all comes down to one question. Am I going to hold out my hand and trust the Lord even
though life isn't fair, even though I have more questions than
answers?'"[55]

Our trust doesn't negate the need to seek God's plans. We
need to discover if He might be willing to reverse our losses. If
so, we follow His leading. If not, we solicit help for acceptance.
We are overcomers, not victims, through the lordship of Jesus.
We wonder what the Lord plans for each of our lives now.

Trusting vs. resting. Maybe it's a matter of resting in God
when healing doesn't happen, rather than just trusting in Him.
It is so comfortable, so peaceful, and so restful for Carole to relax
in the Lord. Strangely, though, she doesn't feel she understands
how to "trust." When she says, "Trust the Lord," she sometimes
adds, "But to do what?" To use this for her good? Or to use it
for His glory? Those seem inadequate reasons for suffering. "To
do what?" Take care of her? He has and will; still, circumstances
don't seem very pleasant. She concludes maybe "resting" is actually
a step further than "trusting." Perhaps it's a deep level of trust,
knowing God is so great she can leave everything to Him; she
can completely rest in Him knowing she's safe.

Concluding Thoughts

For our unending storms, spiritually, we keep coming back to Isaiah 55:8–9. We don't understand why He lets bad things happen to good people, but we know He is always with us. He loves us beyond our comprehension, and so He wouldn't cause us to hurt and wouldn't even allow it, except for some good reason unknown to us. That is why we call it "faith." And this faith brings peace.

In the context of continuing storms, we have seriously considered these questions. Is God trustworthy or not? Yes. Has He been there for us? Yes. Who is He? Our answers: The One and Only True God, loving, righteous, sovereign, all-powerful, and all-knowing. We have examined Jesus' life and considered what He did for people. We have remembered things He has done for us in the past. We have answered the question about who the center of the universe is—God or us. We have considered the claim that God is our crutch. To that, Carole asks, "What can you offer me if there is no God? What will comfort me? What purpose exists for my life? What hope is there for my future since my prognosis is further disability?" Considering all these angles and more, we answer the question "is He worthy to be trusted?" with a resounding "yes!"

FJ's Closing Thoughts for You

"Hello, fellow sojourners who travel through lives of unending storms of discomforting hurt and pain.

"Just finished having morning devotions with that lady I've been hanging around with for more than fifty years. Had a momentary vision as we began to pray, and I felt so relaxed in God's presence. There was total peace—no worry or anxiety, all angst gone. I just rested in the presence of the good Lord above. A vision of an unnumbered multitude of people all lying restfully at ease in God's presence. Today, right now, at this moment of time, in this dangerous, seemingly out-of-control world, people all over the planet are finding and receiving the Holy Spirit's ease of mind and the comfort God imparted to us.

"God's people live far apart yet find they are spiritually invited by Jesus to join the community of faith and have rest in the Lord. Whether working, suffering martyrdom because of faith in God, or being subjected to unending illness, they discover there is rest in the Good Shepherd. Many people have found blessed, all-encompassing, joyful, stress-free, soul-saturating rest in the Lord. We love you and ask this blessing from our Savior God to be yours. This was the message: Jesus sends His love."

Part 3
Responding to Storms—What You Can Do

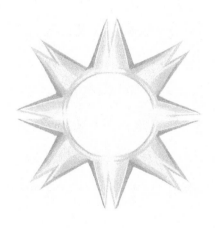

Chapter 16

Watching Others' Storms—
How You Can Help

"Teamwork allows common people to attain
uncommon results."

—Anonymous

FJ and Carole will never forget the generosity and consideration dis-
played by their Ione friends in preparation for Tom's wedding. While
FJ and Carole were traveling to Portland to pick up Tom's fiancée and
bring her to Ione for their upcoming wedding, their friends busied them-
selves at the parsonage. They knew it needed repairs and deep cleaning.
So, the men and women worked together, fixed problem areas, and
super-cleaned the house. FJ, Carole, and Pairum returned to a sparkling
clean home. What a surprise! It sure eased the wedding preparations.

Since, by definition, an invisibly disabled person can't execute
all normal life activities, someone may need to offer aid in
various ways. The primary consideration? Understand your friend.
Is he a private person who doesn't wish to receive help? Respect
that. Private prayer is always an option. Does she need help but

is embarrassed to ask? Consider her needs and tactfully suggest help in specific areas. Or is your friend one who expects help for everything? Decide what is practical for you to do, explaining your reasons, if necessary. Be firm and gently stick to your choice.

Remember that belief and friendship are often what the chronically ill need most. These gifts cost nothing to offer, but they aren't necessarily easy to achieve.

Practical Responses

Only imagination and resources limit how many possibilities of useful actions exist to help those who will accept it. One response could be as simple as acknowledging the person's presence with a "hi." Or as expensive as paying for a housecleaner regularly. Maybe as time-consuming as providing ongoing childcare. And then, the in-between ways to help: arranging transportation for medical care or shopping; housecleaning for a special occasion; contributing limited financial aid; cooking a meal, or filling whatever specific need arises. Don't overlook the simple act of offering friendship.

If you are a caregiver, you both look at and live within the storms. Because you are responsible for the care of another person, you must take excellent care of yourself. Try to eat right. Seek to get enough sleep. Exercise appropriately. Have regular medical checkups and follow the doctor's advice. Heed your emotions; find ways to relieve the pressures. If necessary, obtain respite care for your loved one, so you can relax.

Emotions

At first glance, the area of emotions may appear completely personal and within the individual's control. However, friends and family often provide encouragement, helping the person cope more easily. You can boost your friend's spirits by your support. Offering specific help to their family shows you care. Your presence in person, by phone, or on social media empowers him as he realizes you remember him. Invite her to go out for coffee if she can, or bring a snack to her house, and your action tells her she is important to you. Better yet, if three or four people band together and organize, someone can reach out to the friend every week. How uplifting that would be!

Help your friend laugh. Loan him a comedy to watch. Buy her a joke book. Share memories. Encourage your friend to find humor in everyday life.

These ideas—and others you come up with—go a long way to overcome your friend's isolation. They will lift your friend's mood, lessening depression. One caution: it's unrealistic to expect your friend to always feel and act upbeat. The lives of invisibly disabled people can be difficult and challenging.

One area which demands some type of intervention is suicide. Do you have a valid reason to suspect a close friend is considering this? Talk to him or her or contact a trusted advisor. Don't worry that broaching the subject will make a non-suicidal person consider suicide; experts say it will not. If suicide appears imminent, seek immediate help—a hotline, pastor, or counselor. If the process has already started, call 911. Exercise caution if you don't know the person very well, and be careful regarding your assumptions. Above all, don't gossip about the situation; you may hurt someone's reputation. But since suicide is irreversible with serious repercussions, use your best judgment to help your friend.

You may be able to help your family members or friends as they face fear and worry. Research might help eliminate reasons for these emotions. If you are computer savvy, you could help in this way. If you have a close relationship, you can ask what they fear and look for a way to decrease it. Diminishing fear or worry reduces frustration and anger.

Grief is an integral part of adjusting to life with invisible disabilities. Ron Hall, following his wife's death, stated, "It angered me that people might think some pat little Christian phrase would quench the inferno of my grief. At other times I realized people meant well and, mainly, spoke wounding words because they didn't know what else to say."[56] Yet, your presence in their lives as they cope with loss-caused changes helps them in their grief and sadness. Loss of sight, hearing, or the ability to walk are enormous losses that one likely cannot overcome in a brief time. But the need to grieve is also present in relatively small losses—especially those expected to increase over time. Remember, too, grief can recur even years later. It can pop up again with each new loss.

Acceptance and New Purpose

Accepting limitations and finding new purpose remain personal actions. Again, observers can help or hinder the process. As a caring and compassionate friend, you can offer positive help. Your friend living in inclement weather—whether showers or hurricanes—faces tough changes. He may prefer not to face an unknown future, but at some point, he must. However, exercise care in helping him accept adjustments. Don't force the issue. Alternatively, she may appear to be aggressively adopting her new lifestyle. Beware, she may be covering up grief. Empathize with her and walk with her through these stormy times.

As to finding new purpose, a friend may prove quite valuable. Help him see strengths in his life. Encourage her to look for ways her hobbies could become her new purpose. Exercise patience, be available, and give your dweller friend time to adjust.

Relationships

Family connections. Your own grandparents, parents, siblings, or aunts and uncles may be invisibly disabled. If so, they will benefit from your support. They need your belief and acceptance even more than your friends do. If they live close by, encourage them with visits and support. In long-distance relationships, express love and reassurance through phone calls, emails, social media, or an occasional package.

Humor defuses many troublesome situations. Shared laughter helps each one lower the emotional pain level caused by circumstances beyond their control.

Attempt to help children live as normal a life as possible. Provide respite childcare for a harried parent. If appropriate and needed, offer monetary assistance. Take children on outings. Attend school games and performances.

Be part of a support system. Believe what they tell you (unless you have proof to the contrary). Research their conditions to understand better what they experience. Reassure them of your love. Be aware of their abilities and limitations; don't expect them to act beyond their ability. Respect their independence and allow them to do what they can. Include them in your activities whenever possible.

Comfort for friends. As with words you speak, take care in expressing comfort. The needs of people enduring continual storms differ from those experiencing temporary suffering. Dwellers experience a permanent change in their lives from losses. Family members who are caregivers need comfort, too, for their lives have substantially changed. Sometimes, when appropriate, a hug may bring calm; it expresses acceptance and a variety of emotions. Simple words such as "I know things are difficult for you" convey affirmation and love. On occasion, actions help. Tailor your expressions of comfort to the person's situation; ideas will be limited only by your creativity.

Remember, in deep grief, words may not be needed or appreciated. However, prayers, either unspoken or verbalized, can help. Dostoyevsky reportedly said, "The darker the night, the brighter the stars; the deeper the grief, the closer is God." Advocating an awareness of God supports your suffering friend.

FJ wrote the following prayer in an email to relatives undergoing the beginnings of storms. It serves as an example of comfort.

> Dear precious, heavenly Father: I'm asking for Your divine presence to flood the lives of these loved ones with Your nearness. Please grant them spiritual wisdom and common sense from You; we all have need of such things to be wise and devoted servants to our Savior God. May the Holy Spirit surround our lives completely, and the heaven-sent angels help us in these troubling times. Father, Son, Holy Spirit—Savior God, please cleanse and guide us, for we confess that the Holy Scripture is true. Nothing can succeed apart from You, for all things that are noble, true, and soul-satisfying exist only in the heavenly Father. Abba, thank You for blessing me with a family so wonderful. I just have to love them all the time. Amen.

Thoughtful conversations; caring actions. Words hurt or help others. This is especially true regarding the invisibly disabled. Many sayings carry a different connotation to those who hurt. One useful practice is to try to understand their situation. What would you like to hear someone say? What words might distress you? Words that mean one thing to you could mean the opposite to a dweller. Inflections and body language also convey meaning.

People with hidden limitations often add an implied "but" when they hear the normal compliment, "You're sure looking good today." The dweller may think you are implying they must feel good since they look good. Instead, be specific. "Your hair looks nice today" or "I love the color of that shirt." Maybe, "Isn't your dress new?"

At church, work, or school, you may realize your friend is

back again after an unexplained absence. Please don't say, "Hi, Don. You've been gone. It's been a while." That acknowledges you know he was missing, but Don may hear you saying he just did not want to be there. It's better to say, "Hi Don. Good to see you back again. Glad you're feeling well enough to come today." Thus, you recognize the fact he wasn't there. It also tells him you know he was feeling bad without dwelling on it. When Carole must leave church early, she wishes someone would realize she must be in severe pain and contact her later. To be acknowledged as a real, hurting person—what a blessing and comfort!

When you become aware your friend needs help, there are better ways to offer your aid than the generic expression, "Just call if you need something." Many people in permanent needy circumstances will respond to a general proposal of help with a no because they may—unfairly, perhaps—assume you don't truly mean it, or they just don't know if you have enough time to meet their needs. A specific offer tells the hurting you are serious and lets them know how much you can help.

Again, consider your friend's circumstances. A better approach is to be observant and envision specific help. Does he need a ride? Does she need help to sweep her floors? Do they need childcare, so they can see the doctor together? Does he need to know he is remembered? Contact him by email, phone call, social media, or card, at least occasionally.

You may think those living in Stormyland are being hyper-sensitive, and possibly they are. Alternatively, they may have experienced too many negative interactions. Or possibly, they are just overwhelmed with their problems and find it difficult to function well in social settings.

Churches help. One woman caring for her husband undergoing chemo posted on Facebook regarding her need for housecleaning. Her friend answered, "I am sure you are finding this out, but there needs to be a church-wide push to train people how to care for the caregiver. So much attention is given to the one suffering, but being the prime caregiver is hard and lonely."

Thoughtful church members acknowledge the dweller's existence and personhood. They do this by saying hello and compassionately asking how they are doing. They take the time to listen, letting the person vent if needed, and crying with them when appropriate. Furthermore, they offer prayers according to the person's expressed needs. If able, they seek to help. Sometimes they, or the entire church, can provide financial relief. And remember, teams of people willing to share a load on behalf of a dweller can help in ways limited only by their imagination and creativity.

Medical care. Even in the field of medical care, you, as an observer, might provide aid. Transportation to appointments can be helpful. This saves the working spouse having to take time off. If your friend is single, your help could be critical. If she has surgery, she might appreciate a hospital visit. His family, especially children, may well need care. Perhaps she will need help when she returns home. Many times, government help or insurance is available, but not always, so financial aid might be appreciated. If you have a remarkably close relationship and he's amenable, you might accompany him to see the doctor to help him remember what is said. Only you know your friend and whether he's open to receiving help, but it never hurts to ask.

Healthcare professionals, you can help or hinder the invisibly disabled in coping. Believe what they tell you, clarifying when necessary. Be open with them. Explaining your conclusions and giving them a chance to ask questions helps establish a trusting relationship. Not listening to them, disbelieving what they say, or acting as if you are all-knowing often destroy the patient-practitioner connection.

Spiritual Issues

At first glance, you may wonder how to encourage your friend with spiritual concerns. Of course, prayer comes to mind. Most people appreciate it when someone offers to pray for them; ask for permission first, and inquire as to what they see as their needs. Beyond that, transportation to the church of their choice might be appreciated. Make sure they're physically able to attend, and find out if they have special needs that should be provided for while there. Loans or gifts of DVDs or CDs by favorite artists illustrates another possibility. Buy, lend, or check out books in which your friend is interested. Offer a journal. The key here is knowing your friend.

We leave you with this thought: "A word of encouragement can make the difference between giving up or going on."[57] We extend our heartfelt thanks to all you storm observers who have encouraged and helped us throughout the decades.

Chapter 17

Navigating Your Stormyland—Tips for You

"A killer storm is bearing down on your campsite. The power goes out during an epic snowstorm. Your home and family are threatened by rising floodwaters. When the weather is at its worst, will you be at your best?"
—Dennis Mersereau, *The Extreme Weather Survival Manual*

Carole's Stormyland began suddenly, but several years passed before she realized she would never leave it. During that time, one doctor gave her practical advice, comparing her energy level to having one cup of water for all day. He outlined her choice: drink that cup all at once and have none for the rest of the day, or sip the water, making it last until night. The choice was hers. Carole gradually became aware she could no longer do something whenever and wherever she chose, but with adequate planning, she could still live a fulfilling life.

For our unknown friends who suffer from tempestuous weather, here we'll review the material we've presented. We pray you may discover ideas to help you more easily cope with your storms.

Practical Issues

Principles to maximize limited abilities. Because dwellers can't meet life on normal terms, we must devise practical responses to make the most of our limited abilities. We present five principles that anyone in Stormyland can apply. See if these resonate with you and formulate your specific responses.

1. Know your body, your limitations, and your abilities. Assess your condition. Resist the temptation to push yourself.
2. Assess your circumstances. Redefine expectations. Do only what your strength or condition permits you to do.
3. Evaluate and use your strengths. Harness this power as you learn specific ways to compensate for what you can't do.
4. Accept—or even seek out—help when you need it. Recognize when you really can't do it all and need assistance.
5. Find practical ways to move forward with your life.

Specific actions. If limitations involve fatigability and weakness, focus on energy conservation. When shopping, ride a cart. At meetings, sit rather than stand. If hiking, shorten the distance or use a wheelchair or scooter. Have realistic expectations.

One important practical consideration is your weight. If you must lead an inactive lifestyle, putting on pounds is difficult to avoid. Unfortunately, since many people can't exercise more if they eat that yummy extra, the only option is to not eat it at all. This advice doesn't apply if you have a malfunctioning digestive system.

Learn specific ways to compensate for what you can no longer do. If handwriting is difficult, utilize a computer. Employ assistive devices. Use a wheelchair for hiking or shopping. If blind, obtain the help of a seeing-eye dog. Play games with or read to children by sitting at the table or holding them in your lap. Use a microphone or give up speaking if your voice volume is too low to speak to a group. And don't be afraid to seek help from your local church or other organization.

Find a community of support. If you can't locate local groups, look online. Many websites that exist for learning about invisible disabilities and specific conditions also offer Facebook groups for personal interaction. Look up your disease or disorder on Facebook, and you will likely find a group of people who understand what you face.

For you with severe limitations necessitating spending most—or all—of your time in bed, creativity is a necessity. Search out ideas to keep your mind and spirit sharp. If possible, use a different bed for daytime than for nighttime; a resting place where the family gathers diminishes isolation. Keep a shoebox with necessary items close by your bed—remotes, an intriguing book, Kleenex, encouraging Bible verses, lip balm, notepad and pencil, earbuds, and medicines all fit neatly. Use a phone, tablet, or laptop to keep connected to the world.

Finally, be sure to add fun to your life. Take time for yourself. Choose a de-stressing activity, be it crafts, light yard work, reading a book, or listening to music. You will be happier, and so will your companions.

Emotions

Positive emotions. Amid turmoil and problems, dwellers still enjoy rainbow times and sunbreaks—even if only for minutes or hours. It may be a joke on television, a cute child, or a literal rainbow. It is true: happiness still exists. But you may need to seek diligently for hope, joy, kindness, love, peace, patience, and the faithfulness of others. Search for and concentrate on these constructive emotions.

Faith and hope enable us to recognize these sunbreaks. As one character said, "Faith is what allows us to believe in the beauty behind that dark glass. It's a gift from God, not something we can conjure or create. It's a gift we choose to accept, much like a child opening a box on Christmas morning."[58] Oswald Chambers defines faith well: "Faith is not intelligent understanding, faith is deliberate commitment to a Person where I see no way."[59]

Search for positive words to replace negative ones in your everyday conversation and thought life. Be careful about your attitude. Accept the changes. Discover what brings you happiness. Look back at good memories. Brighten your life by adopting an upbeat outlook.

Gratitude changes the focus to God and others, lessening the desire to complain. A look at life yields reasons to be thankful. Expressing gratitude to those who helped encourages them and you too.

Negative emotions. Various activities can help when fear or worry comes knocking. Try to figure out the reasons for these emotions. Change your focus. Meditate on verses or poetry. Read a book. Listen to helpful or relaxing music. Live one day at a time. Visualize favorite people or places and remember pleasant times. Find humor. Make plans for when angst comes around. Note special songs to listen to. Record positive sayings to focus on. Make a list of relevant verses. Have a list of ten fun activities available.

Neglected fear and worry leads to frustration, which causes anger. Reading books, researching reputable websites, talking with respected friends or trusted advisors, or seeking a counselor are excellent methods of overcoming these troubling emotions.

Depression and thoughts of death may result from physical problems, so check with your doctor. After ruling out a physical cause, see if you are overwhelmed by challenges and limitations. When thinking about death, remember these words: "Prepare for eternal life but work hard in this one. Always."[60] A man who lived with severe dystonia said, "At the end of days that have been extremely difficult and frustrating, I sometimes lay my head on the pillow almost hoping I don't wake up in the morning."[61] However, he thought about joys he would miss, such as watching his grandchildren grow up, and he always came back to being glad for life.

Life on this earth retains value, no matter how difficult it is. If needed, seek help from a dependable person to lessen the stress. Consider engaging in fun, encouraging, or uplifting activities.

Losses and changes. Everyone encounters changes in their lives, and most learn to cope with them. However, for those who live in perpetual nasty weather, coping presents more of a challenge.

If your condition is progressive, continuing losses will be a part of life. Acknowledge and accept this. Remember, finding a new sense of normal is a process that takes time and varies according to the individual's specific conditions and life situation. Along the way, avoid envy of the healthy. Somebody has defined jealousy as the art of counting someone else's blessings. Counteract that emotion by actively looking for satisfying things in your life. Seek help, if needed, to find your new normal.

You can devise plans to counteract negative thoughts and emotions and react proactively. Concentrate on your breathing, relax painful muscles, and refocus your thoughts. On especially challenging days, review your chart of happy memories. Examine and evaluate your to-do list. Apply spiritual applications that worked. Change activity or even plans for the day. Practice positive acceptance. Change negative self-talk to positive words. These strategies may require resourcefulness, which may be hard during difficult times. If you are experiencing new symptoms, see the appropriate doctor, and don't assume your conditions are worsening. Seek positive ways to handle changes, even when challenges become more troublesome.

The desire to spare others' feelings by hiding your problems may be admirable, but masking pain to the point of deliberately concealing it poses a detriment to emotional health—yours and theirs. When people are more than casual acquaintances, they may need to know how you are feeling so they can respond appropriately.

Two extremes exist in a dweller's life. On one end, you may push yourself beyond endurance to prove nothing is wrong. On the other, you may passively accept you can't do anything. This component of coping with changes involves accepting that not everyone will understand.

Acceptance and New Purpose

Most importantly, we need to see ourselves as persons of worth. See the value in our lives. Respect other people, especially those close to us. Grieve losses and work on accepting what is. Then seek new purpose. Prepare by inventorying your talents, how they can be adapted, and what your remaining physical abilities are.

Sam Moss is a good example. She is severely limited and in extreme pain now, but she uses her executive skills to write her wildly successful blog and moderate her Facebook group, bringing encouragement to others' lives.

Relationships

Family. In normal everyday life, relationships with family members are complex, ranging from excellent and full of love to poor and filled with dislike for each other. Families dwelling in storms because of one member's limitations experience the same spectrum of emotions. However, these families' relationships become even more complicated. Consider consulting a family counselor.

Be sure to keep lines of communication open. Honesty and openness—whether with a spouse, children, or extended family—are critical to good relations. Of course, this doesn't excuse whining, bullying, aggressiveness, or unpleasantness. In addition to the basic give-and-take indispensable to satisfactory relationships in normal life, you must find ways to let other family members know what you feel and why without overwhelming them. Find the balance between hiding your pain to spare your family misery and being open about your current feelings so they will understand. How you can accomplish this depends on the personalities involved and the quality of relationships.

Gratitude for help offered encourages the one assisting. Awareness and acknowledgment of caregivers' extra responsibilities can refresh those who give so much.

Friends and social settings. We residents of Stormyland need to be aware of our attitudes. We are often worn out emotionally by our struggles, making it more difficult to function in social situations. It's easy to become hyper-sensitive when fatigue combines with unthinking or insensitive people asking questions or offering help inappropriately. We need to beware of judging others by our circumstances.

Are we too quick to ignore or refuse help because we judge the other person is not serious, or we think they're too busy? Do we get our feelings hurt easily when people ask questions in a manner we deem offensive? Maybe learning better communication skills is our answer.

Perhaps the hardest emotion to bear is loneliness caused by isolation. Whether your disability is blindness, PTSD, weakness, or pain, you likely can't be as socially active as before. Leaving the house can be difficult. Friends could leave you behind as their busy lives continue unchanged. Family members might not be supportive, leaving you out of their activities. It may require ingenuity to overcome the loneliness, as isolation may be unchangeable.

Another opportunity to combat loneliness is to join a support group or a church. You might meet new people who are willing to take the extra effort to be your friend. If it's possible for you, be a help to someone else.

Medical care. Working with medical personnel often constitutes a significant portion of a dweller's time. Carole has learned to stand up for herself. That can be difficult with certain practitioners. Sometimes they're busy and don't wish to take the time, or they may be having a terrible day. Health professionals are well educated, but some may arrogantly believe you have no medical knowledge. Be respectful but stand your ground, especially if it is an important issue. If your doctor won't listen, if he doesn't seem to be knowledgeable, or if she's uninterested in becoming informed about your problems, find another doctor. May you be blessed, as Carole has been, to find an open-minded medical team that accepts her strange symptoms as true.

The patient, or caregiver in some cases, needs to prepare for each appointment. Know what to convey to the doctor about the specific reason for your visit. Do you have new symptoms? Are old symptoms worse? Where is the problem? When did it start? What makes it better or worse? Or do you just need more information to handle your challenge? Carole finds it helpful to make a written list of these items. Prioritize this list if there are many items to cover. Most doctors appreciate this.

Plan a method to remember what the doctor says. Take notes. Or tape the visit, if allowed. A family member or friend who accompanies you could be responsible for recalling specifics.

Evaluate what the practitioner says. You know your body best; be firm. If what he says makes little sense, research further. Talk to others with similar conditions. Speak again to the doctor about your questions or see a different practitioner. Make the best decision possible.

We find it invaluable to keep a list of records: dates of hospitalizations, tests and results, vaccinations, lab results, and doctors' names and addresses. Computers make this easier. This way, you have important information at hand when you see a new doctor or—horrors—if someone loses your records. These records also help you keep your problems in perspective.

Take responsibility for knowing as much as possible about your condition(s). Become informed. Use the internet, but stick to reputable sources like the Mayo Clinic. Look for websites about your problem, especially an association or foundation. For example, the Dystonia Medical Research Foundation is the go-to site for credible information about dystonia. Find support groups in your area. Ask your doctor for sources of more information. The more facts you have, the easier it is to stand up for yourself.

We hope these suggestions enable you to de-stress when relating to the medical community. When you find a good network of practitioners, you might even enjoy the help they can give you.

Spiritual Issues
The perfect start concerning spiritual issues is to seek God for yourself and His plans for you. Searching Scripture helps as you seek God and as you grow in your faith. Reading the Bible or remembering a special verse brings enabling strength for hope and endurance. Make a note of verses that speak to you in special ways. Singing or listening to music is uplifting and soothing. Prayer, talking and listening to God, is another way to grow closer to Him. As we've shared before, a pastor friend once said, "Pray without ceasing and don't cease without praying." If you are able, seek a church where the Bible is taught and people are friendly. Learning and worshiping with like-minded Christians provides another avenue of growth.

A special concern to the invisibly disabled is the question of why God lets things be so hard. The answer is to realize and accept the truth that God's ways are not our ways. You may need to tussle with God about that. In Matthew 11:28–30, Jesus tells us, "Come to Me, all who are weary and heavy-laden, and I will give you rest. Take My yoke upon you and learn from Me, for I am gentle and humble in heart, and YOU WILL FIND REST FOR YOUR SOULS. For My yoke is easy and My burden is light" (emphasis ours). In biblical times, people used yokes for oxen to guide them, making it easier to pull loads. Yokes were custom-made, sanded, and smoothed. Properly made, yokes did not hurt the oxen. Likewise, we trust the custom-made yokes that Jesus makes for us.

In closing this chapter, we leave you with this quote commonly attributed to Winston Churchill: "The pessimist sees difficulty in every opportunity. The optimist sees opportunity in every difficulty." As dwellers in unending storms, we face many difficulties. So, if we are optimists, we see many opportunities for positive outcomes.

Chapter 18

Living Stormy Lives—
Summing Up the Storms

"Deadly tornadoes. Devastating hurricanes. Raging
wildfires. Lightning strikes. Are you prepared
for wild weather?"

—Dennis Mersereau

*FJ, in his chair, and Carole, in her recliner, talk about their experiences
living with invisible disabilities. "These last thirty-five years have
been tough, but we prevailed in what seems like unending storms.
Maybe sharing our difficulties can help someone else thrive in theirs.
Besides, so many people don't understand what life is like for someone
living with unseen limitations. We should write a book."*

*Their Stormyland included a hurricane or two and several severe
thunderstorms in the following eight years, complete with hail and
high winds. FJ underwent five surgeries and three small strokes, each
of which left Carole needing temporary care. Carole's neuromuscular
conditions spiked, causing increased disabilities.*

Stormyland Revisited

Stormyland is an unusual place, unduly familiar to some and unknown to others. Our vision for dwellers, overly accustomed to this place, sees them finding encouragement and more coping strategies. We long for increasing numbers of people untouched by chronic illness to understand the constraints dwellers in Stormyland face daily. We hope some of you, with time and ability, will reach out and help where needed. Our chief desire, along with other residents, is to be acknowledged as individuals and accepted for who we are. Even a "hi" will suffice.

Who is affected? Carole endures neuromuscular and autoimmune disorders. Jayme suffers from digestive and other autoimmune illnesses. Jean experiences severe migraines and multiple other ailments. Gary's cardiovascular disease was terminal. The list continues—Sam's rare bone disease, Jerry's blindness, Wes's Agent Orange. Even more limitations: deafness, mental illness, PTSD, and so many others.

We learned invisible disabilities can strike anyone without regard to age, race, ethnicity, nationality, religion, wealth, or education. The Silent Stalker strikes whoever, wherever, with whatever. He is no respecter of persons.

What is Stormyland like? In short, each person's Stormyland differs. Jayme's landscape is distinct from Jean's and from Carole's. And Gary and Kathy's experience differs from most other residents.

Will it ever end? The title of this book, *Unending Storms*, says it all. No—short of a miracle from God—Stormyland will never end.

Where is it? People in the chronic illness Facebook groups which Carole frequents live all over the world.

Why does it happen? Along with the dwellers in this book, most Stormyland residents never know why they landed there. Some, like Gary, may have made poor lifestyle choices. Veterans such as

Wes are disabled because of war injuries. FJ's arthritis difficulties stem from aging, complicated by diabetes, even though he keeps his well-controlled. He inherited a tendency for strokes, again complicated by diabetes. But others, including Jean, Carole, and Jayme, never learn the source of their difficulties.

Practical, Emotional, and Relational Issues

How can only one book address practical issues for every dweller? Neuromuscular problems, autoimmune diseases, blindness, deafness, and mental health concerns differ substantially. Not to mention the multitude of other invisible disabilities. Therefore, we've only presented what works for us and others with whom we've interacted directly. We just cannot write the largest medical book ever attempted.

At times, many invisibly disabled people need practical help. Compassionate observers can offer this aid. One caution: tread carefully, as some people don't want help even if it's needed.

A trail of confusing symptoms for which modern medicine currently has no answers can be summed up as maddening medical maladies. These disorders confound us since there is no rational logic for them, no known causes, and no cures. As the outlaw in *Big Jake* said, "If it's my fault, your fault, or nobody's fault, the result will be most unfavorable." In this movie, John Wayne portrays Big Jake, whose grandson, Little Jake, was kidnapped by this outlaw and his gang. These words were spoken at the meeting concerning the ransom delivery, but they aptly describe our bewilderment about causes for our imperceptible conditions. How do we live with something we can't understand?

Invisible disabilities seemingly come from nowhere, somewhere, or anywhere. This is akin to our Silent Stalker, who quietly sneaks into a victim's house to take one's possessions. What does this malicious villain do? It removes freedom from pain and sometimes diminishes thought processes. Loss of hope adds to the burden of mental and physical pain. It hinders the will, making it an effort to achieve a purposeful life. Haunting questions linger for some: What is my purpose now? What good can my life contribute to self and society? What use am I?

Losing the feeling of self-worth is a pain in one's soul, eating away the ambition to even keep on existing. How desperately needed is the right friend or supportive spouse. A comforting congregation of kindred spirits brings to the hurting the light of wisdom and the comfort that conveys love and the value of life. Perhaps the most distressful pain comes when no one cares about the disabled. Everyone needs a unique someone who shows them they are special.

Our chronic conditions impact diverse relationships. Family. Friends. Coworkers. Acquaintances. Medical personnel. Despite our challenges, though, we can sustain meaningful connections. It may take work on our part and understanding on theirs, but it is possible.

Sufferers with unending storms of pain find unlikely ways to live meaningful, productive lives. How can storm dwellers make their lives mean something positive? Give of yourself lovingly and sensitively whenever possible. Think of others. Pray for the help you need, then receive graciously and thankfully when others are sensitive to your unique situation.

Many thousands of people not ordinarily associated with the physically stricken continue to be unaware of the variety of needs experienced by those who are invisibly disabled. Millions suffer from work carried out by the unknown Silent Stalker within; countless are the quirks and turns they experience. And so, the mystery of medical maladies mystifies everyone, complicating relationships with family and friends. To maintain the relationship, the observer must recognize and accept the dweller. The Stormyland resident may need to explain realities to the one outside the storms. A complex relationship, indeed.

Spiritual Questions

We rejoice in knowing God doesn't require people to carry out specified feats to earn His approval. Therefore, He welcomes even profoundly disabled people if they love Him completely with their heart, soul, mind, and strength. God calls for us to acknowledge Him as God and ourselves as persons who have wronged Him or other people, thus needing to repent. Once we repent and call on Jesus to save us, we need to love Him with everything within us. Carole, for one, as a weak person who tires quickly, thanks God He is within her reach. Love with heart, mind, soul, and strength. She can do that!

Even amidst our storms, we still choose to assert God is worthy of our trust in this life, and we look forward to heaven. If God doesn't exist, neither does heaven. Thus, our suffering knows no end. What an awful idea! It's beyond endurance to even contemplate the suggestion these pains, weaknesses, and limitations are all there is to our existence. Why live? Yet, God exists. He lives. Therefore, our life has purpose. This absolute trust in God enables us to not only persevere but to have purpose in life.

Carole acknowledges her fundamental spiritual principles as she prays, "You are my peace amidst the unending storms of my life. Knowing You keeps me rational. Trusting that You have a plan—and that it's good in some way—helps me continue keeping on. Believing in You allows a measure of happiness among all the loss, pain, and weakness. Feeling Your presence makes the difference between life and death. Recognizing heaven awaits me—that perfect place of no pain and of relationship with You— brings strength to hold on and hope of joy to come." In addition, she asserts she knows God differently and more deeply than would have been likely without her storms.

Philip Yancey closes his book with his belief: "The problem of pain will have no ultimate solution until God re-creates the earth."[62] For Stormyland dwellers and observers alike, Yancey's further words express our conclusions on the question of God and pain. "My anger about pain has melted mostly for one reason: I have come to know God. He has given me joy and love and happiness and goodness. They have come in unexpected flashes, in the midst of my confused, imperfect world, but they have been enough to convince me that my God is worthy of trust. Knowing Him is worth all enduring."[63]

Our foundational belief remains. We don't desire to know Jesus just because we want to be healed; we long to know God through Jesus because He is Creator, Sustainer, and Redeemer of our lives. He isn't the means to an end; He is the end.

And Finally . . . Forever-Sunny Days in Heaven

No more storms! Sunshine and blue skies! Forever! Heaven will be filled with endless joy. Residents will never say they're dissatisfied or bored. There will be perfect vision, total freedom of movement, and complete strength. Heaven will be filled with eternal comfort, including freedom from pain. All this and unhindered fellowship with Jesus! Living there means fellowship with friendly folks who are perfected with a heavenly nature. The whole population will be filled with the goodness of God.

Everyone there will recognize the Father through Jesus and see Jesus through the Holy Spirit. They will learn this through the Word of God, the Holy Bible. How does one become a resident of heaven? Jesus, the Savior of the world, said in John 3:16, "For God so loved the world that He gave His only begotten Son that whoever believes in Him shall not perish, but have eternal life." To enter heaven is a privilege granted to those who believe in Jesus, Immanuel, God with us. Jesus not only grants eternal life but a purposeful, fulfilling, and joyful life here on earth. Jesus said He is the way, the truth, and the life. This life Jesus spoke of is like living water inside you. All this and heaven too!

Goodbye

And now, we say goodbye. Many of you observers will leave Stormyland. We hope you will visit your local version of this place, bringing cheer and encouragement to those who live there. Unfortunately, we dwellers will never leave Stormyland, but we trust you have found inspiration and helps to navigate your own storms.

It is our hope you have enjoyed this journey as we have explored life with invisible disabilities. May God be with you always.

Appendix

How to Know God—As Easy As A-B-C

Salvation offered by the heavenly Father, the Creator of heaven and earth, is not complicated. According to the Bible, every human has a rebel nature against the way God created people to live; this nature allows storms to form. Humanity's history is one of internal, personal corruption that blinds people to peace, love, and harmony between themselves and their divine Creator. God loves each person. His words, found in His inspired book, the Bible, tell us the Father "is patient with you, not wanting anyone to perish, but everyone to come to repentance" (2 Peter 3:9 NIV).

Why would people perish? some ask. The answer lies in God's nature of perfection. To be clear, this perfection prevents God from creating anything imperfect. He created people to be perfect, to live without any imperfection, to live with all the peace, love, and positive feeling for others that He planned for humanity to have. But people choose to trade away His way of living for a life of failings and shortcomings, and thus come the storms. If the Lord accepted imperfection, then heaven would become populated with imperfect people. Since God could not accept such a place, heaven would no longer exist.

However, God has a plan that will transform us into acceptable inhabitants for His forever-sunny heaven. Jesus took our guilt for sin and the resultant punishment we deserve, dying in our place. Because Jesus died for our sins, He offers to forgive anyone who asks Him. But Jesus did not stay dead: He became alive again. He has the power to give victory over the death we all as sinners deserve. He is the only one who can offer eternal life to all who believe He is God's only Son. This begins the moment a person seeks peace with God. To receive peace with God for all time, just use the simple ABC acronym to talk to God in your own words.

A—Admit the Weather's Bad

Admit you are not living as the Bible admonishes people to. Romans 3:23 demonstrates that every individual has done wrong. In a nutshell, just realize you are a sinner rebelling against God. The bad news is that the penalty for sin is eternal death, as described in the first part of Romans 6:23: "For the wages of sin is death."

B—Believe the Weather-Maker

And now the good news. Believe Jesus Christ came as God incarnate, fully God and fully man, and that as the only sinless person to ever live, He could pay the penalty for our wrongs. The last part of Romans 6:23 gives us the good news: "But the gift of God is eternal life in Christ Jesus our Lord." So God leaves us with hope, but receiving that hope requires a choice from you. "For God so loved the world that he gave his one and only Son, that whoever believes in him shall not perish but have eternal life" John 3:16 (NIV).

C—Choose to Live a Sunny Forever

Choose to ask the Savior God, the only true God, to forgive you for being a sinner: a rebel against God, resisting faith in Jesus as Savior. Confess that your sinful nature is more than you can conquer, and you desire the Lord God to change and free you from sin and guilt. He will bring eternal life to you.

These ABCs lead you to the answer that Jesus prayed in John 17:3, "Now this is eternal life: that they may know you, the only true God, and Jesus Christ, whom you have sent" (NIV).

Now you have the answer to "How can we know God?"

Glossary of Medical Terms

acetaminophen. Brand name is Tylenol.

activities of daily living (ADL). These include six basic activities: eating, bathing, dressing, toileting, walking, and continence.

aneurysm, cerebral. Abnormal bulge or ballooning in the wall of a blood vessel. It can burst and cause internal bleeding and even death. Cerebral refers to the location, the brain.

autoimmune disease. Overactive immune system that attacks and damages its own tissues.

Botox (botulinum neurotoxin). Neurotoxic protein used therapeutically to treat cervical dystonia and other conditions. Injected into spasmed muscles, it blocks the neurotransmitter, acetylcholine, which, in turn, reduces or eliminates excessive muscle contractions. Each affected muscle needs an injection. It wears off in three months and must be repeated.

cervical dystonia. See dystonia.

chronic fatigue syndrome (ME/CFS). Debilitating disorder whose main symptom is extreme fatigue that does not respond to rest and is not caused by any other medical condition. Alternatives names are myalgic encephalomyelitis (ME) or systemic exertion intolerance disease (SEID). Since there are no tests specific to CFS, it can be difficult to diagnose although symptoms can be treated.

co-morbidity. Medically, it refers to a person having a primary disease or disorder plus one or more additional diseases or disorders.

costochondritis. Inflammation of the cartilage in the rib cage.

Crohn's disease. Inflammatory bowel disease, causing inflammation of the digestive tract. Different areas of the digestive system can be affected. This inflammation often spreads deep into the layers of affected bowel tissue, which can be painful and debilitating, sometimes leading to life-threatening complications. Symptoms can be mild to severe and include abdominal pain, severe diarrhea, fatigue, weight loss, and malnutrition. It cannot be cured, only treated.

deep brain stimulation (DBS). Brain surgery allowing electrodes to be implanted to deliver electrical impulses, which block or control abnormal activity. It is mostly performed for Parkinson's but is also used for dystonia, tremors, and epilepsy. The person uses a handheld programmer device to control the electrodes and turn them off and on.

degenerative arthritis. Chronic disorder damaging cartilage and tissues surrounding a joint. It is also called osteoarthritis, degenerative disc disease, and wear-and-tear arthritis. It causes stiffness, pain, and joint malformation. It usually occurs in older adults. It is different than rheumatoid arthritis.

discectomy. Spinal surgery to remove a ruptured (herniated) disc. A disc is the cushion sitting between two vertebrae; it acts like a shock absorber allowing bending and movement without pain. If the disc material presses on a nerve root or spinal cord, it causes pain, weakness, or numbness.

dysphagia. Difficulty or discomfort in swallowing. Dysphagia can be as mild as feeling a lump in the throat or as serious as the inability to swallow. Aspirating food is possible. Neurological disorders, including stroke, are a common cause.

dysphagia, oropharyngeal. Symptoms include the inability to control food or saliva in the mouth, difficulty initiating a swallow, choking, coughing, frequent pneumonia, and reflux.

dystonia. Movement disorder causing muscles in the body to contract and spasm involuntarily. Individuals affected by dystonia cannot control or predict the movement of their bodies. Symptoms of dystonia manifest differently in every patient. Dystonia may affect a specific part of the body or many parts simultaneously. Major types of dystonia include cervical dystonia (neck/shoulder); spasmodic dysphonia (speaking); blepharospasm (eyelids); oromandibular dystonia (face, jaw, tongue); limb dystonia (hand/arm or foot/leg); and generalized dystonia (many parts simultaneously). Commonly treated with Botox every three months.

EKG (electrocardiogram). Test to check for heart disease. It records the electrical activity of the heart through electrodes attached to the chest.

exacerbation. Increase in the severity of a disease, its signs, or symptoms.

fatigability. Medical condition in which muscles become weaker after minor exertion due to a decline in their ability to generate force. A long period of time, sometimes days, may be required for muscles to regain full function. This condition occurs in several neurological diseases.

fibromyalgia. Disorder characterized by widespread musculoskeletal pain accompanied by fatigue, along with sleep, memory, and mood issues.

fusion. Major spinal surgery that joins two or more vertebrae by means of inserting bone or bone-like material to prevent unwanted movement. The surgeon uses metal plates, screws, and rods to stabilize the vertebrae. Reasons for this operation include misalignment of the spine, severe degenerative disc disease, spinal instability, or fracture. This surgery is used only when all other options have failed.

gastroenterologist. Doctor specializing in the health of the digestive system.

gastroparesis. Weakness of muscles of the stomach, or the nerves controlling those muscles. It causes mild to severe digestive problems. Another name for it is *slow stomach*.

glaucoma. Group of eye conditions that damage the optic nerve and cause loss of vision. If left untreated, it can cause blindness. Lost vision cannot be restored. Regular eye exams can catch it early.

idiopathic rare bone disease. Believed to result from a mutant gene. In Sam Moss's case, it results in her bones thickening and becoming deformed. This greatly increases the chances of her bones breaking; they often do not heal.

irritable bowel syndrome (IBS). Common chronic disorder affecting the large intestine. Symptoms include cramping, abdominal pain, bloating, gas, and diarrhea or constipation, or both.

laminectomy. Spinal surgery that removes the lamina (back part of a vertebra covering the spinal canal) to enlarge the spinal canal. This removes pressure on the spinal cord or nerve. Bone spurs and ligaments may also be removed. This problem is commonly caused by arthritis or aging. This surgery is used when more conservative treatments have failed.

lancinating. Causing stabbing or piercing sensations.

laryngospasms. Vocal cord spasm. It limits air passage through the larynx, making it difficult, or even impossible, to talk or breathe. It starts suddenly and can be frightening because of breathing issues. However, it is not life-threatening; it just feels like it. Breathing ability returns when the spasm releases.

Lou Gehrig's disease. Also known as amyotrophic lateral sclerosis (ALS). This progressive neurodegenerative disease affects nerve cells and the brain and spinal cord. As motor neurons degenerate, they die, leaving the person unable to initiate accompanying movement. The motor nerves affected by ALS controls voluntary movement and muscle control. Currently, it is terminal.

lupus. Systemic autoimmune disease. Lupus-caused inflammation can affect many parts of the body, including joints, skin, kidneys, blood cells, brain, heart, and lungs. There is no cure for this difficult-to-diagnose disease, but treatments but are available to decrease symptoms.

migraine. Chronic neurological disease disproportionately affecting women. It is more than just a severe headache. It affects men and children too. Symptoms and frequency differ for each person, as does treatment. Rare forms can defy successful treatment. In its severe forms, it is disabling.

modified barium swallow. Test using fluoroscopy to show actual swallows in real-time. It is used to diagnose swallowing difficulties. Another name is Video Fluoroscopic Swallowing Exam (VFSE).

multiple sclerosis (MS). Abnormal response of the body's immune system directed against the central nervous system (CNS). CNS includes the brain, spinal cord, and optic nerves.

neurogenic bladder. Name given to a number of urinary conditions in people who lack *bladder* control due to a brain, spinal cord, or nerve problem. A high risk exists for serious complications.

neurological. Anything having to do with the nerves or the nervous system. Includes the anatomy, functions, and organic disorders of nerves and the nervous system.

neurologist. Doctor specializing in disorders of the nervous system. This includes diseases and disorders of the brain, nerves, muscles, and spine.

neuromuscular. Anything that pertains to or affects both muscles and nerves.

paresis. Weakness of voluntary movement. Incomplete paralysis. Partial loss of voluntary movement. Impaired movement.

paroxysmal nonkinesigenic dyskinesia [or dystonia] (PNKD). Episodic movement disorders in which abnormal movements are present only during attacks. *Paroxysmal* indicates that symptoms are noticeable only at certain times. *Nonkinesigenic* relates to an episode not triggered by sudden movement.

Dyskinesia or *dystonia* broadly refers to movements of the body that are involuntary. Between attacks, most people are generally neurologically normal, and there is no loss of consciousness during the attacks. It is a rare disorder.

physiatrist (PMR). Doctor who works to restore optimal function to people who have injured muscles, bones, tissues, or nervous system.

plantar fasciitis. Inflammation of the fascia in the foot causing stabbing pain. It is more common in runners, but risk factors include age, obesity, and improper shoes. Another cause is an abnormal pattern of walking, which can stem from neurological disorders.

post-polio syndrome (PPS). New condition affecting survivors of polio decades after the acute illness of polio. Major symptoms are pain, fatigue, and weakness. New weakness is considered the hallmark of post-polio syndrome. Less common symptoms are new sleep/breathing/swallowing problems. Some survivors experience muscle atrophy or muscle wasting.

post-traumatic stress disorder (PTSD). Serious condition caused by experiencing or witnessing a terrifying event of actual or threatened physical harm. It can be lasting and serious enough to interfere with normal life activities. This is a common occurrence from trauma that occurs in a war zone but can also happen following other types of trauma.

psoriatic arthritis. Form of inflammatory arthritis sometimes afflicting people who have psoriasis. Joint pain, stiffness, and swelling can affect any part of the body, including fingertips and spine. These symptoms range from mild to severe and may flare and remit. Untreated, this disease can become disabling.

Raynaud's disease. Vascular disease, causing cold toes and fingers due to spasms of blood vessels. It also rarely affects the lips, nose, or ears.

remission. Disappearance of the signs or symptoms of a disease. It can be temporary or permanent.

rheumatoid arthritis. Autoimmune disease that affects the lining of the joints causing pain, swelling, bone erosion, and joint deformity. The inflammation produced can damage other parts of the body.

rheumatologist. Doctor specializing in non-surgical treatment of rheumatic (autoimmune and inflammatory) illnesses, especially arthritis.

Sjögren's syndrome. Systemic autoimmune disease that primarily presents with dryness of mouth, eyes, and skin. It can cause profound fatigue. It can affect any organ in the body: the kidneys, gastrointestinal system, blood vessels, lungs, liver, pancreas, and the central nervous system. It often occurs with rheumatoid arthritis, lupus, or scleroderma. It increases the risk of lymphoma. Symptoms can be mild or debilitating; they can remain steady, worsen, or occasionally get better.

small fiber neuropathy. Occurs from damage to the small unmyelinated peripheral nerve fibers present in skin, peripheral nerves, and organs resulting in pain.

"spells." Carole's name for her unusual disorder. One doctor compares "spells" to PNKD, though there are differences. Severe loss of function—partial paralysis—usually accompanied by sleep and pain characterizes a "spell." In the first stage, Carole begins to relax, often sleeping and experiencing only mild, if any, pain. This lasts ten to fifteen minutes, and if interrupted, Carole experiences neither relaxation nor discomfort. During stage two, her legs (and sometimes her arms or front of her head) feel "encased," bringing mild to severe pain. This part lasts fifteen to forty-five minutes. If the "spell" is disrupted by noise (phone ringing, person talking, shoe dropping), the pain increases and recovery takes several hours. Regaining function begins in stage three, which can be the most painful. As the pain recedes, the muscles slowly return to normal. This stage is the longest, at thirty to sixty minutes or more. Stopping the "spell" increases pain and lengthens the recovery time. An entire episode totals thirty minutes to two hours.

stress test, exercise stress test, or treadmill test. Shows how the heart works during physical activity and reveals problems with the heart's blood flow. Heart rhythm, blood flow, and breathing are monitored during exercise on a treadmill or stationary bike. Alternatively, a drug that mimics exercise can be given. This test diagnoses coronary artery disease or heart rhythm problems and guides the treatment of heart disorders.

TENS unit (transcutaneous electrical nerve stimulation). Uses electrical stimulation to block pain signals to underlying nerves. Electrodes are applied to the body and attached by wires to the control unit. Electrodes are placed and removed every day.

traumatic brain injury (TBI). Injury resulting from a severe blow or jolt to the head. It can affect any aspect of a person's life, including personality and mental abilities. Brain injuries do not heal as other types do, although people can recover the ability to function in life. TBI manifests in various ways in different individuals.

Endnotes

Introduction

1 "Americans with Disabilities: 2010" (July 2012), 4, accessed May 11, 2017, https://www.census.gov/content/dam/Census/library/publications/2012/demo/p70-131.pdf. (page discontinued). The Survey of Income and Program Participation data collected in 2010 showed 38.3 million severely disabled people, 15.2 million of whom used wheelchairs, canes, or walkers, leaving 23.1 million severely disabled persons whose disabilities are not easily discerned.

2 F. Marcus Brown, III, "Inside Every Chronic Patient Is an Acute Patient Wondering What Happened," Journal of Clinical Psychology-In Session, Volume 58 (November 2002): 1444, Wiley Periodicals, Inc. Quoted in Connell and Connell, But You LOOK Good, 33.

3 Definition of disability from the Social Security Act, 42 U.S.C. §423(d) (1).

4 "Disabilities Affect One-Fifth of All Americans," Census Brief (December 1997), 1, accessed May 19, 2018, https://www.census.gov/prod/3/97pubs/cenbr975.pdf.

5 "What is an Invisible Disability?" Invisible Disabilities Association, accessed May 10, 2017, https://invisibledisabilities.org/what-is-an-invisible-disability/.

6 Wayne Connell and Sheri Connell, *But You LOOK Good* (Parker, CO: The Invisible Disabilities Advocate, 2009), viii.

7 Henry Drummond, quoted in L.B. Cowman, "Streams in the Desert" (Grand Rapids, MI: Zondervan, 1977), June 13.

Chapter 3

8 For more information about the unusual phenomenon Carole calls "spells," see the glossary.

Chapter 4

9 Martin Pistorius, *Ghost Boy* (Nashville, TN: Nelson Books, 2013), 111.

10 Edgar Page Stites, "Trusting Jesus," (hymn) 1876.

Chapter 5
11 Philip Yancey, *Where Is God When It Hurts?*, rev. and expanded (Grand Rapids, MI: Zondervan, 1990), 211.
12 Christine Miserandino, "The Spoon Theory," *But You Don't Look Sick*, accessed March 8, 2018, https://butyoudontlooksick.com/articles/written-by-christine/the-spoon-theory/.

Chapter 6
13 Paula Dumas, "7 Types of Migraine: Which Do You Have?," Migraine Again, July 17, 2019, https://migraineagain.com/10-types-of-migraine-which-do-you-have/.
14 Operation Heal Our Patriots: A Project of Samaritans Purse, season VII (Boone, NC: Samaritan's Purse, 2018), 17.

Chapter 7
15 Jeffrey H. Boyd, *Being Sick Well: Joyful Living Despite Chronic Illness* (Grand Rapids, MI: Baker Books, 2005), 58.
16 Ron Hall and Denver Moore, *What Difference Do It Make?: Stories of Hope and Healing* (Nashville, TN: Thomas Nelson, 2009), 79.

Chapter 8
17 Max Lucado, *Fearless: Imagine Your Life Without Fear* (Nashville, TN: Thomas Nelson, 2009), 74.
18 Jerry Sittser, *A Grace Disguised: How the Soul Grows Through Loss* (Grand Rapids, MI: Zondervan, 2004), 24.
19 Martin Pistorius, *Ghost Boy: The Miraculous Escape of a Misdiagnosed Boy Trapped Inside His Own Body* (Nashville, TN: Nelson Books, 2013), 34.
20 Lee Strobel, *The Case for Grace: A Journalist Explores the Evidence of Transformed Lives* (Grand Rapids, MI: Zondervan, 2015), 168.
21 Langston Hughes, *The Collected Works of Langston Hughes: Essays on Art, Race, Politics, and World Affairs* (Columbia, MO: University of Missouri Press, 2002), 525.

Chapter 9

22 Jerry Sittser, *A Grace Disguised: How the Soul Grows Through Loss* (Grand Rapids, MI: Zondervan, 2004), 198.

23 Bill Crowder, "Test Match," *Our Daily Bread,* July 2016, July 25.

24 Lee Strobel, *The Case for Grace: A Journalist Explores the Evidence of Transformed Lives,* (Grand Rapids, MI: Zondervan, 2015), 168.

25 Sam Moss, *My Medical Musings,* "Old Loves, New Loves," February 1, 2020, https://mymedmusings.com/2020/02/01/old-loves-new-loves/?fbclid=IwAR3c-GQPWMARKocgPnvM-joIe4m0l5FyO7kjhLIkBUk8S3ZYSufxYW0Q16hA.

26 Philip Yancey, *Where Is God When It Hurts?,* rev. and expanded (Grand Rapids, MI: Zondervan, 1990), 206.

Chapter 10

27 Erin Prater, "Chronic Illness in Marriage," Focus on the Family. January 1, 2008. https://www.focusonthefamily.com/marriage/chronic-illness-in-marriage/.

28 Barry J. Jacobs, "When Caregivers Fall Out of Love," AARP, July 31, 2017, https://www.aarp.org/caregiving/life-balance/info-2017/spousal-caregiving-divorce-fd.html.

29 Jerry Sittser, *A Grace Disguised: How the Soul Grows Through Loss* (Grand Rapids, MI: Zondervan, 2004), 36.

30 Wayne Connell and Sherri Connell, *But You LOOK Good: A Guide to Understanding and Encouraging People Living with Chronic Illness and Pain* (Parker, CO: The Invisible Disabilities Advocate, 2009), 49.

Chapter 11

31 "Horse or Zebra? Determining if You are Dealing With a Rare Diagnosis," Thrive AP (website), June 18, 2013, https://thriveap.com/blog/horse-or-zebra-determining-if-you-are-dealing-rare-diagnosis.

32 Kate Mitchell, "Chronically Ill Tips: What To Do When a Doctor Isn't Listening to You," *Kate the {Almost} Great,* May 24, 2019, https://katethealmostgreat.com/chronically-ill-tips-when-a-doctor-isnt-listening/.

33 Mitchell, "Chronically Ill Tips."

34 Mitchell, "Chronically Ill Tips."

Chapter 12

35 Ed Young, "Overcoming Tough Times: How NOT to Comfort," (sermon), *The Winning Walk*, broadcast in February 2014.

36 Philip Yancey, *Where Is God When It Hurts?*, rev. and expanded (Grand Rapids, MI: Zondervan, ©1990), 2009. 233.

37 Yancey, 210–213.

38 Yancey, 234–235.

39 Wayne Connell and Sherri Connell, *But You LOOK Good: A Guide to Understanding and Encouraging People Living with Chronic Illness and Pain* (Parker, CO: The Invisible Disabilities Advocate, 2009), 47.

Chapter 13

40 Lee Strobel, *"The Case for Miracles"* (Grand Rapids, MI: Zondervan, 2018), 253.

41 Sam Moss, "Not All Stories Can Be Champagne and Roses," *Medical Musings with Friends,* November 20, 2019, accessed April 9, 2020, https://mymedmusings.com/2019/11/20/not-all-stories-can-be-champagne-and-roses/?fbclid=IwAR1sSVqdPmFRmFCybCMy3ZBr4_C6agBrB4eeO8Z-VK5ZXVfKX9OeiPj3qWIk.

42 Sam Moss, *My Medical Musings.*

43 Patricia Rushford, *Red Sky in Mourning: A Helen Bradley Mystery, Book Two* (Ada, MI: Bethany House Publishers, 1997), 167.

Chapter 14

44 L. B. Cowman, comp., *Streams in the Desert: 366 Daily Devotional Readings,* edited by James Reimann (Grand Rapids, MI: Zondervan, 1997), March 23.

45 Lysa Terkeurst, *It's Not Supposed to Be This Way,* (Nashville, TN: Nelson Books, 2018), xiii.

46 Lisa Harris, *Vanishing Point* (Grand Rapids, MI: Revell, 2017), Adobe Digital Editions EPUB file, 226.

47 Ralph O. Muncaster, *Why Does God Allow Suffering* (Eugene, OR: Harvest House Publishers, 2001), 33.

48 Dee Henderson, *The Healer* (Carol Stream, IL: Tyndale House Publishers, 2002), Adobe Digital Editions EPUB file, 66.

Chapter 15

49 Edward Mote, "The Solid Rock," (hymn) ca. 1834.

50 Philip Yancey, *Where Is God When It Hurts?*, rev. and expanded (Grand Rapids, MI: Zondervan, 1990), 222.

51 Abraham Lincoln, *Lincoln's Devotional* (Great Neck, NY: Channel Press, 1957), xv.

52 Bruce Goldman, "Stunning Details of Brain Connections Revealed," Science Daily, November 17, 2010, https://www.sciencedaily.com/releases/2010/11/101117121803.htm, Accessed March 18, 2020.

53 Frank Harber, *Beyond a Reasonable Doubt: Convincing Evidence for Christianity* (Lynchburg, VA: Liberty House Publishers, 1996), 17.

54 Wendell Berry, "The Peace of Wild Things," quoted in Philip Yancey, *Prayer: Does It Make Any Difference?* (Grand Rapids, MI: Zondervan, 2006), 21.

55 Tina M. Radcliffe, *Mending the Doctor's Heart* (Ontario, Canada: Harlequin, 2013), Adobe Digital Editions EPUB file, 61.

Chapter 16

56 Ron Hall and Denver Moore, *What Difference Do It Make?* (Nashville, TN: Thomas Nelson, 2009), 79.

57 Richard DeHaan, "Dying for Encouragement," in *Our Daily Bread: Daily Readings from the Popular Devotional, Vol. 2* (Grand Rapids, MI: Discovery House Publishers, 2009), March 4.

Chapter 17

58 Victoria Bylin, *Until I found You* (Minneapolis, MN: Bethany House, 2014), 300.

59 Oswald Chambers, *The Quotable Oswald Chambers* (Grand Rapids, MI: Discovery House, 2011), 238.

60 Worth, Lenora, *Bayou Sweetheart* in January 2014, bundle 2 of 2. (Ontario, Canada: Harlequin Books, 2014), Adobe Digital Editions EPUB file, 129.

61 Mike Beck, *Living in a Body with a Mind of Its' Own: The Emotional Journey of Dystonia* (Bloomington, IN: Author House, 2013), 41.

Chapter 18

62 Philip Yancey, *Where Is God When It Hurts?*, rev. and expanded (Grand Rapids, MI: Zondervan, 1990), 260.

63 Yancey, 260.

Recommended Resources

Books

Boyd, Jeffrey H. *Being Sick Well: Joyful Living Despite Chronic Illness.* Grand Rapids, MI: Baker Books, 2005. (Encouraging ideas by the author whose wife was very sick. Includes stories of other people also.)

Cerveny, Randy. *Freaks of the Storms: From Flying Cows to Stealing Thunder.* New York: Thunder's Mouth Press, 2006. (Interesting book about unusual weather phenomena.)

Connell, Wayne and Sherri Connell. *But You LOOK Good: A Guide to Understanding and Encouraging People Living with Chronic Illness and Pain.* Parker, CO: The Invisible Disabilities Advocate, 2009. (Excellent resource about living with invisible disabilities. Very helpful in explaining to others what life is like.)

Cowman, L.B., comp., *Streams in the Desert: 366 Daily Devotional Readings.* Edited by James Reimann. Grand Rapids, MI: Zondervan, 1997. (Devotional book, first published in 1925, that still speaks to people today, especially those living in storms.)

Open Windows: A Guide for Personal Devotions. Nashville, TN: Life-Way Christian Resources. (A daily devotional magazine published quarterly.)

Our Daily Bread: Daily Readings from the Popular Devotional, Vol. 2. Grand Rapids, MI: Discovery House Publishers, 2009. (Daily devotionals presented monthly, the best of which are compiled in annual books.)

Pistorius, Martin. *The Ghost Boy: The Miraculous Escape of a Misdiagnosed Boy Trapped Inside His Own Body.* Nashville, TN: Nelson Books, 2013. (Autobiography of Pistorius' struggles as a boy horribly misdiagnosed. Continues through his adult years as he overcomes immense obstacles.)

269

Sittser, Jerry. *A Grace Disguised: How the Soul Grows Through Loss.* Grand Rapids, MI: Zondervan, 2004. (A must-read about suffering and how to overcome it by a man who lost his mother, wife, and daughter in one traffic accident.)

Terkeurst, Lysa. *It's Not Supposed to Be This Way.* Nashville, TN: Nelson Books, 2018. (Biographical account of the author's difficulties in life and strategies to overcome them.)

Yancey, Philip. *Where Is God When It Hurts?* Rev. and expanded. Grand Rapids, MI: Zondervan, 1990. (Classic study of the subject of pain and God. Excellent source to help understand why God might allow pain.)

Organizations

Invisible Disabilities Association. https://invisibledisabilities.org/ (Organization advocating for those with invisible disabilities.)

Joni and Friends. https://www.joniandfriends.org/ (Organization ministering to disabled people nationally and internationally.)

National Suicide Prevention Hotline. 1-800-273-8255. (Someone is always available by phone 24/7 to answer questions or provide help.)

Websites and Blogs

Griffitts, Carole. Navigating the Storms. https://www.navigatingthestorms.com/. (Website providing hope, help, and information for and about those living with invisible disabilities.)

Moss, Sam. *My Medical Musings.* https://mymedmusings.com/ (Blog and podcast loaded with insights and hope gleaned from Sam's life living with her rare bone disease.)

Rest Ministries. http://restministries.com/ (Website specializing in information and devotions for people with chronic conditions. Has a section with advice on how to form local support groups called HopeKeepers.)

About the Authors

Before the storms, FJ and Carole and their sons, Tom and Bill, lived a typical life. After serving four years in the Air Force, FJ pursued education, graduating college and seminary. For fun, they walked around the neighborhood, played soccer, drove through scenic areas, hiked, and camped. From then to now, their family has enjoyed togetherness as it expanded to include two daughters-in-law and seven grandchildren.

FJ and Carole live in the Pacific Northwest, where they continue delighting in the outdoors, albeit on a limited scale. FJ walks the nearby lakeside trail, soaking up nature. Occasionally, Carole accompanies him on her scooter. Camping adventures continue as they visit mountains and beaches. Tom and Bill also live close enough for frequent get-togethers, at one home or another. Young adult grandchildren add zest to life.

After seminary, FJ served as pastor and Army Reserve Chaplain, counseling, writing, and speaking. In 2015, Carole started a website, Navigating the Storms, for invisibly disabled people and those who care about them. She connects with others through Facebook groups where they chat about writing, owning and managing websites, and navigating life with chronic illnesses. She has spoken to health profession students.

FJ and Carole can be reached through their website, Sunbreaks, where they have photos highlighting stories of their family. You can put faces to names and see how their family has grown.

www.sunbreaksbooks.com

Thanks for reading *Sunbreaks in Unending Storms*! If you were helped by the book or have learned about people who live with invisible disabilities, we would really appreciate a short review as this helps new readers find this book.

Made in the USA
Monee, IL
30 July 2021

74609822R00177